CW00502005

Keto Adapted

Your Guide to Accelerated Weight Loss and Healthy Healing

Maria Emmerich

Keto Adapted

Copyright © 2013 by Maria Emmerich

All rights reserved. No part of this book may be reproduced or transmitted in any form or by any means without written permission of the author.

ISBN 9781494742645

Published by Maria and Craig Emmerich, printed by Thomson Shore.

Dedication

I once heard someone say, "If you want to hear God laugh, tell him what you have planned!" That statement couldn't have been more true for the past few years of my life. I was totally a planner, and the more I tried to control how things happened, the more frustrated I got. My husband lost his job, my job as a rock-climbing guide didn't pay the bills and we struggled to start our family. All of these trials helped push me in the right direction to my nutrition business. Throughout this journey I have been able to befriend some amazing people that I need to thank.

Jamie Schultz: I remember when you first approached me, "Maria, I love your book, but you need a new cover!" Your photography is incredible! Thank you for the covers of all of my books! I also want to thank you for helping me start my blog; it helped me get up in the morning when I was going through the most difficult time in my life!

Kristen Demulling: To my beloved BodyPump instructor. I remember when you first started teaching class and you looked so young I thought you were freshly out of high school. When you started talking about your daughter in 4th grade my jaw hit the floor! I should have guessed you were a keto-adapted woman! You look wonderful! Thank you for helping with the content of the book.

Nicole Howard: Even though we live so far apart, I still feel so connected with you. I really appreciate you taking time out of your busy schedule to proof read my chapters and ideas.

Emily Derr: You copy editing is truely amazing. Thank you for all your hard work.

Dr. William Davis: Thank you for taking the time to write my forward. Your work is amazing and you are a true role model for me. You have done more to help my family that I could have ever asked for. Thank you!

Dr. David Perlmutter: Thank you for taking time from your busy schedule to write about my book. Your work is really leading science to new places for brain health.

Craig: To my love and best friend. Without your technical skills, patience, editing, encouragement and APPETITE, none of this would have happened. Thank you for never complaining when the kitchen is a disaster after a recipe photo shoot, or the dishwasher is stacked with dishes in a way they will never get clean, when the laundry isn't done or the kids need a bath because I am swamped with work. I am so lucky to have a husband like you who jumps into helping without any complaints. SHMILY.

Contents

Foreward

By William Davis, MD and David
Perlmutter, MD

M aria Emmerich has done it again.

      In her quest to help readers understand how to regain ideal health, wellness, and weight, Maria has developed a unique talent to deliver the nuts and bolts of a healthy nutrition program. In her newest effort, Keto Adapted, she clears up much of the confusion over the ultra low-carb lifestyle and why it is superior for overall health and weight.

For years, we were terrified of ketosis, the metabolic state generated when virtually no carbohydrates are available for energy. Metabolic ketosis was often confused with ketoacidosis, a dangerous condition that type 1 diabetics typically have before their condition is diagnosed because insulin is unavailable to allow glucose to enter the cells of the body. While both conditions do indeed involve ketone production, it came to be recognized that diabetic ketoacidosis involved orders of magnitude greater levels of ketones, far above the naturally adaptive levels of metabolic ketosis.

There have been observations made over the years that hinted at the advantages of metabolic ketosis. We've known, for instance, that children with intractable seizures unresponsive to medicine, or even surgery, respond to a ketotic diet, often with dramatic relief. We've also heard anecdotes of cancers disappearing with extended metabolic ketosis. After all, the method of PET scanning to detect cancer employs a radioactive form of glucose, reflecting the fact that cancers take up more glucose than normal tissues.

What has taken many of us by surprise more recently is that ketosis, i.e., this adaptive state that allows humans to survive—thrive—on a diet minus carbohydrates yet still extract energy from food, provides unexpected advantages in health outside of these unique situations. Not only does ketosis powerfully facilitate weight loss from visceral fat stores, it is also associated with heightened states of mental clarity, reversal of insulin and leptin resistance, and may indeed create a situation that essentially starves cancer cells of their preferred nutrient, glucose.

Maria's Keto Adapted is an approachable, user-friendly discussion detailing how to put the concepts of metabolic ketosis into practice in the context of an overall program to regain and maintain ideal health.

Of course, nothing Maria produces wouldn't be complete without her signature beautiful and delicious grain-free, strict low-carb recipes! Maria is a genuine master of this art. The recipes she provides in Keto Adapted are those that help facilitate a lifestyle crafted to maintain this metabolic advantage.

Maria Emmerich has done an outstanding job creating a user friendly guide to the life changing ketogenic diet. This book will certainly change the lives of many in an incredibly positive way.

William Davis, MD

Author of New York Times Bestseller, Wheat Belly - Lose the Wheat, Lose the Weight, and Find Your Path Back to Health.

Maria Emmerich has done an outstanding job creating a user friendly guide to the life changing ketogenic diet. This book will certainly change the lives of many in an incredibly positive way.

—David Perlmutter, MD

Author of New York Times Bestseller, Grain Brain - The Surprising Truth About Wheat, Carbs and Sugar, Your Brain's Silent Killers.

Chapter 1

Introduction

Throughout this book, I start my chapters with before-and-after photos and testimonial from a former client. These are to inspire you and to give you the motivation to succeed. Some of my clients don't show as much on the outside (weight loss), but their insides (moods, pain, gastrointestinal problems, etc.) are drastically improved. This is the miracle of eating a well-formulated keto-adapted diet: you heal on the inside and the outside, and feel better than ever. Make sure to take your "before" photo before you begin!

Below are my before-and-after photos. Before, I had IBS (Irritable Bowel Syndrome), acid reflux, mood swings, low energy and much more. Now, I have never felt better or had more energy!

—Maria

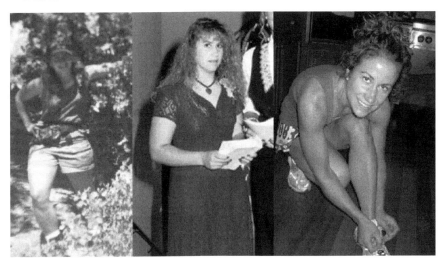

When my dog, Teva, started losing her hair in patches, the first thing my veterinarian asked me was, "What are you feeding her?" Yes! What a good question! But you know what? I have never been asked that question at the doctor. Not once. Not even when I was a teenager suffering from IBS and acid reflux. I was just given a prescription. Nothing frustrates me more than getting a Band-Aid for the symptoms and not addressing the underlying cause of my issues. The prescription doesn't fix what is causing the problem, it only covers up the symptoms. If you also want to start treating the cause of your health problems (not just the symptoms), this book is for you! I have written this book to help you understand where you may be going wrong with your grain- and sugar-free lifestyle. I have over ten years of experience addressing the causes of clients' problems, and this book explains what works!

Let's look at a hypothetical situation: It is Monday morning, and you are running late. You have already begun your grain-free lifestyle so, as you run out the door, you grab a gluten-free granola bar made with dried fruit and nuts.

No time for breakfast means no time to pack your lunch either, so you run to the health food store to grab a gluten-free quinoa and beet salad with kombucha (a fermented beverage for digestive health) to drink. Meetings at work run late, so you nosh on a banana to tide you over until dinner.

Dinner wasn't planned either. Since the whole family is relying on you to prepare dinner, you stop on the way home for an organic roast chicken with mashed potatoes.

Does this sound like you? Are you feeling better with your diet, but the scale isn't moving? Well, of course it isn't. You are still a sugar burner. You may be reading this and thinking, "There was no sugar in this day of eating." Look again. It was *filled* with sugar. "Complex carbohydrates" (such as whole grains and root vegetables) are just glucose molecules hooked together in a long chain. The digestive tract breaks it down into glucose … also known as sugar!

The dried fruit in the granola bar is glorified candy. The quinoa from the salad is a starch that becomes about 9 teaspoons of sugar in your blood for just 1 cup. Though did you really just have 1 cup? Probably not. The beets are also sugar. One cup of cooked beets become another 3 teaspoons of sugar in your blood. Am I driving you nuts? I hope so, because if you are eating "clean" and still frustrated with your weight, you must realize which foods are becoming sugar in your blood.

Sugar is demonized on television commercials and in health magazines (and rightly so), but these critics take a wrong turn when they recommend eating a banana when you have a sugar craving. Guess what? Your sugar craving may have gone away, but only because you ate sugar! Bananas are sweet for a reason. It is the same with kombucha; it tastes sweet because there is sugar in it.

No, a banana isn't the same as eating a Kit Kat bar; however, the prevailing definition of insanity is to keep doing the same thing over and over again and expecting a different outcome. I'm not judging you: I was guilty of this myself. I would eat dried prunes for lunch thinking they were "fat free" and filled with fiber (to keep me full). How brilliant was I? Fifty-pounds-over-weight brilliant; that's how smart I was!

Maybe you read that example and thought, I don't eat that way. I know that diet is way too high in carbohydrates for me. Well, let's dive into another typical day of "healthy" eating that I hear in my office. I had a client come in the other day who described what her diet was on "good" days, and it was still not a fat-burning diet. On "good" days, she took the time to make an egg-white omelet with two organic chicken sausages for breakfast; for a snack, she had eighteen homemade raw-vegan nut-flour crackers; lunch was sautéed turkey in chicken broth; and dinner was chicken with a ton of low-starch vegetables. Puzzled? She was eating way too much protein for her body, which was keeping her a sugar burner. She also didn't eat any healthy fats. As well, she often had "bad" days of eating because the cravings got the best of her. After hearing about her diet, it was no wonder to me why her hair was falling out.

I asked a group of women who have read my book, *Secrets to a Healthy Metabolism*, if they thought the book was suggesting a high protein diet: they all answered yes. This is why I felt the need to write this book. In this previous book of mine, I wrote about how we need to cut out starch and grains, but most people mistakenly replaced those calories with protein. I know this sounds crazy, but you cannot store protein; when you eat too much, it turns into sugar in your blood via gluconeogenesis, a topic which we will dive into in chapter 2.

When I first wrote *Secrets to a Healthy Metabolism*, I was following the tips outlined in this book, but I was afraid readers would think I was crazy if I told them to focus on eating more fat. So as I wrote and consulted with clients, I was quite reserved, gave passive modifications and suggested to take new "baby steps" each week. After years of consulting, however, I have heard the pain in clients' voices. I understand now that most people want an assertive, Jillian Michaels–type approach. So now, I want to step up the plan, tell you to "rip off the Band-Aid" and start adopting a keto-adapted lifestyle now! You deserve this!

There are too many myths about low-carb diets. Everyone knows that sugar is bad for us, but most people don't know what foods turn into sugar. Often times people follow a low-carb diet and complain of unpleasant side effects. In the following chapters, I will explain why this is happening and how to keep it from happening to you. I will refer to the plan I have laid out in this book as a "well-formulated keto-adapted diet" (I will expand on this in the following chapter).

Low-carb diets often get bad press, and many times studies show that they "don't work." Why is this? Well, let us dive into the so-called "low carb" studies. In these studies, the participants were reducing their carbohydrates to 150 grams per day and didn't eliminate gluten or dairy (why that is so important I will explain later). Sure, reducing their carbohydrates from 300 grams a day makes 150 grams look like low-carb, but it isn't! A well-formulated keto-adapted diet will be closer to 30 grams of carbohydrates per day. Cutting out these "complex carbohydrates," as well as gluten, is essential in order for you to become the keto-adapted fat burner we all strive to be.

I am often asked if my methods are considered "Paleo," and if so, why don't I use honey? My answer is no, this is not Paleo. I love all eating practices that eliminate processed foods, and in the past, I would have considered myself a Paleo nutritionist. After a couple years of seeing debilitating ailments not being cured with my Paleo approach, however, I knew there had to be a better way to heal my clients. I always followed a keto-adapted diet myself, but I was more passive in my approach with clients. I thought, Of course they can eat spaghetti squash; they *were* eating white pasta, so changing to the squash would be fine. But in many cases, insulin resistance and inflammation were still issues. My clients' metabolisms were too damaged to handle that amount of starch. Sure, our ancestors most likely could eat the root vegetables and more starch than the clients I see today, but our ancestors did not eat foods like we do today. After all our years of consuming "food" filled with fructose, food dye, MSG, pesticides, and all the other chemicals found in foods today, we need a stricter approach because our cells are so damaged.

My approach is not Paleo because I do not believe that we are meant to live off of lean proteins, a belief that the majority of Paleo books preach. This is not a high-protein diet because too much protein turns into sugar through gluconeogenesis.

The following testimonial is from a client with a diabetic husband:

This past June, my then thirty-eight-year-old husband was in a health crisis. He is a type 2 diabetic who had just developed high blood pressure. His blood pressure was so high, and his weight almost three hundred pounds, that our new family doctor went through the roof. My husband was on the verge of a stroke or a heart attack. He also suffers from severe sleep apnea.

I started us on a diet back then which used lean protein shakes. When I learned about you, I switched over to "your way," now known as the "Maria way" or the "ME way" [ME as in Maria Emmerich] of high fat, moderate protein, and low carb.

Almost a year down the road and he's lost fifty pounds, his blood pressure is much better, and his diabetes is under control. He had a sleep study done, and his very severe sleep apnea is now moderate when he sleeps on his side and only severe if he sleeps on his back. I also have lost fifty pounds, and that's even after spending three months this spring and summer in bed with a broken ankle after a freak ice storm this past April.

We aren't perfect at following [your approach] yet, but we've already made such huge strides forward. We are working at changing the habits of a lifetime. So happy to have found you!

—*Sherrilee*

Sure, there are people who can eat a Paleo diet filled with sweet potatoes and fruit and not be over weight, but this doesn't mean they are healthy. I have had a handful of clients who were female, 115 pounds and had very high blood sugar levels and had to be put on insulin. Not only should diabetics and people who want to lose weight limit their carbohydrate intake, and also limit protein, but everyone should. We are all, in an evolutionary sense, predisposed to becoming diabetic. I want to take you through how fat is stored, but more importantly, I want to demonstrate how we become at risk for diabetes and heart disease.

Let's begin with how weight gain and inflammation happens, starting with our mouth:

1. After you eat excess carbohydrates and/or too much protein, your blood glucose stays at a higher level longer because the glucose can't make it into the cells of the muscles. This toxic level of glucose is like tar in the bloodstream clogging arteries, binding with proteins to form damaging AGEs (advanced glycation end-products) and causing inflammation.

This high level of glucose causes triglycerides to go up, increasing your risk for coronary artery disease.

2. Starch and sugar get stored as fat. (Remember, starch is just glucose molecules hooked together in a long chain, and the digestive track breaks it down into glucose. So, a sugary diet and a starch diet are the same thing.) Because the muscle cells basically have a crust over top of them (called glycation), the cells aren't getting glycogen and are therefore considered "resistant." Additionally, since insulin stops the production of the fat-burning enzyme lipase, now you can't even burn *stored* fat! You can workout all you want, but if you continue to eat oatmeal before your workouts, you will never be a fat-burner: you will remain a sugar-burner and you will continue to get fatter until eventually, those fat cells become resistant too.

3. If the above information isn't bad enough, I have more bad news: insulin levels continue to stay at a higher level longer because the pancreas mistakenly believes, "if a little is not working, more is better." This is *not good*. Insulin is very toxic at high levels, causing cellular damage, cancers, plaque buildup in the arteries (which is why diabetics are more likely to have heart disease) as well as many other inflammatory issues such as nerve damage and pain in the extremities. Starch and sugar destroy nerve tissue, causing tingling and retinopathy, which in turn cause glaucoma and cause you to lose your eyesight.

4. Sorry, but I have more bad news … Our cells become so damaged after a life of cereal and skim milk for breakfast that not only does insulin resistance block glucose from entering muscle cells, but the crust we have formed over our cells also blocks amino acids from entering. Amino acids are the building blocks for our muscles that are found in protein. So now, you can't even maintain your muscles. If that isn't bad enough, your muscles become cannibals. Because your body thinks there is not enough stored sugar in the cells, it sends signals to start to

consume valuable muscles to make more glucose (sugar). You get fatter and you lose muscle.

5. Instead of feeling energetic after you eat, you feel tired, and you crave more carbohydrates. Since you now have less muscle, exercise is getting too darn difficult, and the sad cycle continues.

6. Now comes even more bad news: because of everything your body has been through up to this point, thyroid disorders can occur. When your liver becomes insulin resistant, it can't convert thyroid hormone T4 into the T3, so you get those unexplained "thyroid problems" which continue to lower your energy and your metabolism.

If you don't want any of this to happen to you, there is good news! Here are some steps you can take to avoid the consequences of sugar and starch:

1. Lower your carbohydrates, moderate your protein intake, and increase healthy fats. Do it not only for yourself, but for your kids, too! It is important they don't end up as insulin sensitive as we are.

2. Exercise. I'm not referring to exercise for calorie expenditure, but for hormone control. Even if you are simply walking after meals, your body will benefit. Moving has a major impact on improving insulin sensitivity since muscles burn your stored glycogen as fuel during and after your workout. People mistakenly think that they need to exercise to create a calorie deficit in order to lose weight. This is not how exercise helps with weight loss. Exercise builds muscle, and muscle builds mitochondria. It is in the mitochondria where fat is oxidized so you can keep your cells and your liver insulin sensitized.

When I wrote my first book, I should have named it something other than *Secrets to a Healthy Metabolism*. A "healthy" metabolism is different than a "fast" metabolism. I was obviously referring to a fast metabolism, but a fast metabolism isn't actually "healthy." In our Paleo days, those with a fast metabolism were the "unhealthy" people who died young. But today, they are the people who tell me that they do not have to diet or watch what they eat because they are thin and "healthy." Really? You have no complaints about your health? No ailments that bother you? Just because you are thin does not give you permission to eat sugar and starch in abundance. The higher a person's metabolism is, the more calories are needed to maintain weight. This most likely translates into that person consuming more food than someone with a slow metabolism. While eating more is not a health issue in and of itself, more often than not it means a person is eating less healthy foods than someone who has always struggled with weight. These unhealthy sugary and starchy foods increase risk for metabolic syndrome, and they also increase risk for cardiovascular issues, diabetes, Alzheimer's, joint pain, and inflammation. So even if you are not overweight, this book is for you, too.

Inflammation is the stem of all disease. I hear from many people that they are on an "anti-inflammatory" diet, but are they really? Do they think that since they cut out "sugar" and replaced their sugar cravings with fruit, that it is "anti-inflammatory"? Sure, someone with a healthy metabolism and no inflammation may be able to handle more fruit than someone with chronic pain, but why even stimulate those sugary taste buds? An inflammatory diet is cutting out all sugar and when I say sugar, I also mean starch.

You may be wondering, what's left to eat? No starch, and limited protein? Well, you can eat fat, and lots of it. It is considered a ketogenic diet. You will start to hear more and more information about ketogenic diets and the powerful healing benefits they have. The Eating Academy (a research group lead by Gary Taubes and Dr. Peter Attia) is researching the effects of true ketogenic diets. I write "true" ketogenic diets, because in the past, low-carb diet studies really weren't "low carb" and were often times not well formulated. Sure they were lower in carbohydrates than the recommended 300 grams a day, but even lowering to 150 grams a day is not ketogenic nor low carb in my definition. Another flaw in the studies is that they were still low fat and too high in protein. Also, many of the studies lasted two weeks or less, which is not enough time for the subjects to become keto-adapted.

In this book, I will be giving suggestions for supplements to heal certain ailments that have worked wonders for my clients. Please always check with your primary health care provider before starting any supplement regime. More importantly, it is critical to monitor your numbers and levels of which medication you are on, be it acid reflux medication, insulin, thyroid medication, or blood pressure medication. With this diet and with specific supplements, you will begin to heal; most of my clients no longer need medications. Work with your doctor to monitor your levels and adjust medications accordingly.

So get your "before" photo ready, because in a month, you will be shocked at the difference in your body, inside and out.

Chapter 2

Keto Adaption with Pure Protein and Fat

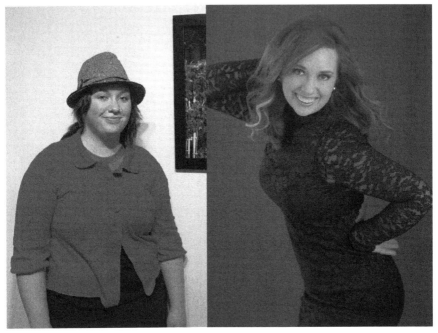

Maria, I have tried so many diets in the past. I will admit I was one to be fooled into thinking that the popular "low fat" diet was the way to go. I can certainly agree with you and say that it's not! After cutting fat and calories from my diet, I found myself losing weight (one pound a week if I worked out a lot). Eventually, though, I would feel deprived and depressed, and gain it all back. In addition, I was noticing my hair thinning a ton! I started seeing my doctor about my hair thinning over a year ago. She did a blood panel and then sent me to see multiple specialists. I've probably had one appointment every couple of months for a year, and still I have no answers; I haven't been directed to take action in any way either. That is what really tipped me over the edge to contact you, Maria. I figured I've already spent so much time and money not *getting any answers. Why not try your way? What have I got to lose?*

From our first email, I could tell that you cared enough to help me. As soon as I booked a session with you, we took action (unlike the doctors office). I listened to everything you said and, well, you helped me change my life. Everything you teach just made sense to me and really "clicked." I started the "Maria way" in October 2012, and it is now January 2013. Since then, I've lost over thirty pounds and I'm still losing!

The most important part for me is that all of the symptoms I had when I came to you are gone or are very close to gone. Anxiety = gone. Hunger spikes = gone. Stress levels = greatly reduced. Not to mention, my hair is growing in thicker, healthier, and much faster. My skin looks amazing, too, and I've been getting so many compliments about it :) Overall, I feel like a million bucks! From the bottom of my heart, thank you!

—Molly

A "Well-Formulated" Pure Protein and Fat Diet

I used to really enjoy sitting and reading women's health and fitness magazines. But since my children came into my life, those days are put on pause (at least until my kids are no longer demanding toddlers who prefer to sit on my lap whenever I open a book). I cherish these times, so I don't mind the interruptions. I did happen to pick up a Women's Health magazine while I was waiting for a weight-lifting class at my local fitness center, and I was shocked that I ever wasted my time reading them. Not only did they push "healthy" whole grains, but they also pushed lean proteins. No fat was included anywhere. This is the so-called clean diet that so many people succumb to in order to try to lose weight. Fat is essential to our diet: our brain and our cells are over 60 percent fat![1,2]

Too many clients of mine remain slaves to the belief that glucose is the only source of fuel for our bodies. Because of this inaccurate belief, they live their lives in fear of running low on glucose. The truth is that fat is the ideal energy source and has been for most of human evolution. We actually need only minimal amounts of glucose, most or all of which can be supplied by the liver as needed on a daily basis. The simple, sad fact that carbohydrates (carbs) and glucose are so readily available and cheap today doesn't mean that we should depend on them as a primary source of fuel or revere them so highly. In fact, it is this blind allegiance to the "carb paradigm" that has driven so many of us to experience the vast array of metabolic problems that threaten to overwhelm our health care system. I can't believe that there is still a large segment of the so-called health and fitness community that defend carbohydrates and glucose as fuel sources with such tenacity.

There are two sources for fuel: you can burn fat (ketone bodies) or you can burn sugar (glucose). Being a fat burner is referred to as being keto-adapted, and it is the preferred metabolic state of the human body. It is why we have all this fat on our bodies, and it is an awesome source of fuel! To understand what it means to be in this preferred state of ketosis, it is useful to examine what it means to be a sugar burner.

What Does It Mean to Be a Sugar Burner?

1. A sugar burner can't easily access stored fat for energy. That means that your muscles cannot oxidize fat when you are a sugar burner. I know, I know, the Runner's Magazine you are reading says you burn glucose for energy, which is why marathoners eat a huge pasta dinner the night before and have oatmeal for breakfast. I did that for years and ran some pretty good marathons, but I was overweight and had lots of joint pain. I essentially wanted a glucose IV drip hooked up to my veins because I was always hungry or "hangry" (hungry and angry). When I was a sugar burner and would go two, three, or four hours without food, or even—dare I say it—would skip a meal, you needed to watch out ... I was "hangry." I was the definition of a suffering sugar burner.

   Our bodies have evolved to depend on beta oxidation of fat for the majority of our energy needs. In a keto-adapted body, fat tissue releases a bunch of fatty acids 4 to 6 hours after eating and during fasting, because your muscles should be able to oxidize them. But since I kept eating bananas, granola bars, and carbs when I would get "hangry," my cells were burning sugar and not fat. Once my blood sugar was all used up, hunger would set in, and my hand would grab for yet another banana.

2. A sugar burner cannot process the fat you eat for energy. The detrimental side effect of this fact is that more fat is stored than burned. Unfortunately, sugar burners end up gaining lots of body fat. A low ratio of fat-to-carbohydrate oxidation is a solid predictor of future weight gain.

3. A sugar burner relies on a short-lived source of fuel for energy. You can only store about 50–90 grams of glucose in your liver for energy conversion, which really isn't a lot. You can also store glucose in your muscles, a process that varies a lot from person to person (trained athletes usually have larger storage sites if they train with carbohydrates). You can't store very much of it, however, unless you count the grams of glucose in the snacks that are in your pockets. For example, let's imagine a very lean man with 12% body fat who is 160 pounds. He has over 19 pounds of fat to burn for oxidation, but the amount of glucose in his muscle and liver glycogens is limited to about 500 grams. Think about this for a second: would you rather have 19 pounds (8618 grams) of energy or 500 grams of energy? I'm choosing the longer lasting energy source.

4. A sugar burner uses up their glycogen stores rapidly during exercise. Whenever I run the Twin Cities Marathon, I love the "wall" we all hit at mile twenty. This feeling is similar to "the wall" that the sugar burner–runners are experiencing. The glycogen stores are pretty much depleted by mile twenty. This is where many runners start to walk. I remember this pain and exhaustion quite vividly; it is hard to forget the great pain and determination that it took to keep going. As a former marathon sugar burner, I wasted my glycogen on efforts where fat would have be able to keep me going.

What Does It Mean to Be Keto-Adapted?

1. Keto-adapted means you can effectively oxidize dietary fat, as well as stored fat, for energy. If you are keto-adapted, your postprandial fat

oxidation will be increased, and therefore a lesser amount of fat will be stored in adipose tissue. Instead, the fat will be used for energy. Basically, fat is now your fuel source (instead of glucose), so your body will readily use your dietary fat for fuel instead of storing it in your body. Your body can also easily switch between burning dietary fat and storing fat for fuel.

2. Keto-adapted (or fat-adapted) means you can rely more on fat for energy during exercise, which means sparing glycogen for when you really need it. Being able to mobilize and oxidize stored fat during exercise reduces an athlete's reliance on glycogen. This helps athletes save the glycogen (which your body can make from protein, too) for the truly intense segments of a session, and burn more body fat. If you can handle exercising without having to consume carbohydrates, you are most likely keto-adapted. If you can perform a quality workout in a fasted state, you are definitely fat-adapted. When fully keto-adapted, your muscles will actually become more insulin resistant as they prefer ketones (the by-products for fat oxidation) for fuel and will leave the glucose for other parts of the body that need it more, like the brain. You can even store ketone bodies in your muscle for future use, just like you can with glucose.

3. Keto-adapted means you have plenty of accessible energy, even if you are lean. If you are keto-adapted, the genes associated with fat metabolism will be unrestrained in your muscles. You have essentially reprogrammed your cells' fuel source.

4. Keto-adapted means you can burn stored fat for energy throughout the day. If you can handle intermittent fasting, can skip a meal, and are able to go hours without getting "hangry" or craving carbohydrates, you are likely keto-adapted.

5. Keto-adapted means you are able to burn glucose if it is available and necessary, but a sugar burner has no choice; they can't flip back and forth. This is why a sugar burner hits a wall during the day and may

need a nap. Being keto-adapted means metabolic flexibility. Keto-adaption allows you to empty glycogen stores through intense exercise, refill those stores, burn any consumed fat that isn't stored, and easily access and oxidize the fat that is stored when it is needed. This enables you to exercise in a fasted state. But since glucose is toxic in the blood, we'll always want to burn it first — then a keto-adapted person can start burning fat. Sugar burners get exhausted and need more sugar because their bodies don't have the ability to switch back and forth. This isn't a suggestion to start adding tons of carbohydrates once you are fat-adapted. Doing so will take you out of ketosis. Fuel your body with fat!

This is not a diet, it is a lifestyle. By eating this way, you will begin to heal your cells (less sugar means less glycation; there will be more on this in chapter on fructose). You will keep transforming into the happy and healthy person you want to be. It took me years to heal my cells: it wasn't something that happened in a month, but with time, my leptin resistance went away.

Leptin resistance is an issue I see with almost every client. After years of eating a low-fat, carbohydrate-rich diet, our cells become resistant to the hormone leptin. This explains why when you eat large amounts of food, you never get the sense of feeling full, a state you might experience when you first adopt a well-formulated keto-adapted diet. With time, however, this diet will heal your leptin receptors, and soon enough you will be full and satisfied for very long periods of time. I never thought that two meals a day would ever be enough for me. But when you eat a high-fat, moderate-protein, low-carb diet, your insulin levels stay nice and even. Hunger happens when your blood sugar dips too low. By never letting it get too high, you avoid the big insulin spike that makes your blood sugar go too low.

There is a home test for measuring your ketones and for determining if you are keto-adapted (more on that at the end of this chapter). If you don't have a ketone tester, then it is more about how you feel. Things like low satiety after eating, hunger a few hours after eating, waking up in the night because of low blood sugar, impaired fat burning, and carbohydrate cravings are all signs of a sugar burner. You can also test your ratio of carbon dioxide you produce to the oxygen you intake to see if you are keto-adapted, but it isn't really practical or possible at home. An RQ (respiratory quotient) of over 1+ signifies that you are burning sugar; if you have a RQ of 0.7 that would signify fat burning. If you are around 0.8, that would mean you are somewhat keto-adapted or in the process of becoming keto-adapted. Clients with high body fat and diabetes have higher RQs. People who are night owls and are nighttime eaters also have higher RQs and low-fat oxidation rates. The good news is that you can change your fate!

Instead of trying to figure out your RQ (or if you don't have a home ketone tester), ask yourself a few questions to determine if you are truly keto-adapted:

1. Can you exercise without eating beforehand?

2. Can you go longer than three hours without eating?

3. Do you have enough energy throughout the day?

4. Do you need a nap in the afternoon?

5. Do you have "brain fog"?

6. Do you have headaches?

7. Do you wake up in the middle of the night hungry?

8. Do you experience "hanger" (hunger and anger)?

If you answered "yes" to the first three questions and "no" to the last five, you are definitely keto-adapted.

> **HELPFUL TIP:** Breakfast isn't the most important meal of the day. "Breaking your fast" is when your most important meal of the day is, whether that is lunch, etc.

Becoming Keto-Adapted

So what does this diet look like? It is an extremely low-carb, moderate-protein, high-fat diet. Do not get this confused with the popular high-protein diets. Too much protein will also become sugar in the blood, just like too many carbs will. The best way to become keto-adapted is to add more fat to your diet. Salt is also essential in restoring energy, which sounds goofy, but I will discuss it in more detail later in this chapter.

The first obvious step to being keto-adapted is to cut out sugar, and when I say sugar, I also mean starch. Complex carbohydrates are just glucose molecules hooked together in a long chain. The digestive tract breaks it down into glucose (just like it does with sugar). So a complex-carbohydrate diet filled with sweet potatoes (or whatever starch you desire) is also considered a sugary diet. To become keto-adapted, you need to start using ketones for energy, not glucose (either from sugar, carbs, or excess protein).

If you are wondering what ketones are, they are a by-product of fat oxidation. Sounds great, right? It happens in the liver during beta-oxidation. Fatty acids are broken down into acetyl-CoA. Acetyl-CoA is then oxidized, and its energy is used for the production of ATP (adenosine triphosphate), the coenzyme used as an energy carrier in the cells of all known organisms — the body's energy source. If excess acetyl-CoA is produced or inadequate quantities of a required precursor called oxaloacetate are present, the extra acetyl-CoA is transformed into ketone bodies. So you can actually produce ketones and oxidize fat for ATP at the same time. We all naturally go through a mild ketosis (nutritional ketosis is what being keto-adapted is called, using fat for fuel instead of glucose) after fasting during a long night of sleep, if you don't eat right before bed and after you've woken up. You need to not eat for over ten hours to be in mild ketosis.

To start producing ketones, my first suggestion is to start with a diet of less than 10 grams of carbohydrates a day. This may seem like an awful battle that you can't win, but it really isn't so bad. Through my passion of cooking, I have developed bread-like foods that I can consume instead. I eat them with fatty meats and spoonfuls of coconut oil in order to fill my cells with the proper percentage of these macronutrients. My favorite breakfast is my protein "bread" dipped (or should I say drenched!) in my organic hollandaise sauce. I often pass my poached eggs to my husband Craig in order to eat more hollandaise. I understand that my protein bread does not taste like French Meadow Bakery baguettes, but add a ton of organic butter to it and you will want to become keto-adapted, too! You will feel so good that you will never again look at those baguettes with a longing desire.

One question I get all the time from clients is, "How much protein is too much?" Well, everyone has a different tolerance, just like with carbohydrates. I work with lots of extreme diabetics who can't eat more than 60 grams of protein a day (about 20 grams at each meal) or they will be kicked out of ketosis. In order to become keto-adapted, you need to turn up your healthy fat intake to push yourself over the adaptation divide as quickly as possible. The amount of fat you need to eat in grams per day will depend on your caloric needs. The following is a good equation to determine the amount of fat in grams you need to consume: Fat grams = (calories * (0.8 to 0.7)) / 9. For example, if you are shooting for 1400 calories a day with 80% of those calories coming from fat intake, then (1400 * 0.8) / 9 = 124 g of fat a day.

If you don't like fatty cuts of meat, you can add medium-chain triglycerides (MCTs) to your diet. MCTs are mainly comprised of medium-chain fatty acids. MCT oils go directly to the liver to be converted into acetyl-CoA for energy and do not show up in cell membranes or adipose tissue. The acetyl-CoA to ATP pathway becomes overwhelmed, which causes the creation of ketones. Consuming MCT oils increases ketone production.

Medium-chain triglycerides (MCTs) are different than long-chain triglycerides. MCTs are absorbed more like carbohydrates and are used and burned quickly by the body; they are not stored in the fat cells, and any extra are converted into ketones. This is why I am very specific with my food recommendations, even with the salad dressings my clients use. It is always best to make your own dressing (and easy, too), but more so because I make it with MCTs rather than with olive oil (or other vegetable oils) which is a long-chain triglyceride and will not turn into ketones for fat burning.[3] Instead of using long-chain triglycerides, which do go into cell membranes and can show up in adipose tissue, MCT oils are less likely to overwhelm the liver's ability to make ATP. It is therefore better to switch to using coconut oil and animal fats.

> **HELPFUL TIP:** If you don't like the taste of coconut, use expeller pressed coconut oil, which does not have a coconut flavor.

MCTs passively diffuse from the GI (gastrointestinal) tract to the portal system (longer fatty acids are absorbed into the lymphatic system) without requirement for modification like long-chain fatty acids or very-long-chain fatty acids. In addition, MCTs do not require bile salts for digestion. Patients that have malnutrition or malabsorption syndromes are treated with MCTs because they do not require energy for absorption, utilization, or storage.[4] MCTs will speed up the ketone production process. On rare occasions, MCT oils have caused nausea in some of my clients if they take too much of it, so be cautious and start out slowly.

MCT oils:

1. ORGANIC BUTTER. According to the nutritional experts and authors of *Nourishing Traditions*, Sally Fallon and Mary G. Enig, PhD, fresh butter is one of the best sources of fat and MCTs. About 12 to 15% of butter is made up of short- and medium-chain fatty acids, according to these authors. This is the type of fat that can be used quickly by the human body for energy. Fresh butter, according to *Nourishing Traditions*, has both antifungal and antitumor properties.[5]

2. COCONUT OIL. Coconut oil contains about 60% medium-chain fatty acids.

3. MCT OIL. Usually derived from coconut oil. Contains about 90–100% medium-chain fatty acids. (used in my Super Salad Dressing recipe).

> **SUPPLEMENT TIP:** There are some supplements that can help you achieve keto-adaptation faster, such as l-carnitine and CoQ10. L-carnitine is an amino acid which aids the breakdown of calories by shuttling fatty acids into the mitochondria, which is our 'fat-burning powerhouse' in our cells where fat oxidation takes place. CoQ10 helps build more mitochondria in your cells. So together, these two supplements help increase the rate of which you become a fat-burner.

One of the best side effects of becoming keto-adapted is the disappearance of the desire for carbohydrates and sugar, but it can take some time. If you find yourself gravitating towards carbs on the weekends, whether it is a beer or a piece of pizza, cheating will stop you from becoming keto-adapted. This is why I often discuss with my clients the possibility of adding in bifidobacteria, 5-HTP, magnesium, liquid zinc, L-glutamine, and other supplements to help deter those nasty cravings that can sometimes get the best of us. Those cravings set me back for years! I would do well during the week, but then I would give in to those cravings on the weekend. I never was truly keto-adapted until I added in supplements to help get rid of those cravings and to stay the course.

Some other common and bothersome symptoms experienced by my clients just starting a keto-adapted diet are headaches, dizzy spells, light-headedness, fatigue, and cramping. These symptoms aren't experienced by all of my clients, but when they do happen, there are some nutrients that can help. This is why I often say a "well-formulated" low-carb diet: when you don't get enough salt or minerals, uncomfortable side effects can occur.

Sodium and Electrolytes

When you have metabolic syndrome, it means you have a lot of insulin circulating in your blood for most of the time. You don't need to be overweight for this to happen. I have had clients who were underweight and still had extreme blood sugar issues. This excess insulin does many wicked things to your body. In the book *Why We Get Fat,* Gary Taubes demonstrates how excess insulin makes you store fat in your fat cells. We focus on that one undesired side effect because we can see its results externally, but the more harmful effects are actually happening internally. Excess insulin also activates the kidneys to retain fluid. I had one client who was extremely obese and would fluctuate up to twenty pounds daily because of water retention. Yep, twenty pounds of water retention! She was experiencing pitting edema in her lower legs.

To test if you also have pitting edema, press your finger into the tissue of your shin bone. If your finger leaves an indentation (basically your finger print), you have pitting edema. Most obese clients complain of this sensation late in the afternoon or after being on their feet all day. What's happening is the excess water retention gathers in the lower legs and soaks into the soft tissues. During sleep, when the body is horizontal through the night, the fluid is redistributed into the upper body. Come morning, the pitting edema has gone away, but then returns as the day goes on. This happens to anyone with insulin issues — it is just more noticeable in those who are overweight.

When clients first adapt to the keto-adapted lifestyle, one of the first side effects is a rapid improvement in insulin sensitivity. Eating low-carb causes insulin levels fall quickly, and your body starts to banish insulin resistance. As insulin levels fall, the kidneys begin to promptly release fluid. One common complaint I get from clients when they first adopt this lifestyle is that they are up in the middle of the night urinating more than usual. This will go away eventually, which is a good thing, but there is also some bad news that comes along with it.

The good news is that when you release that excess fluid, fat oxidation becomes easier. The bad news is that as the extra water goes, it also removes essential sodium and electrolytes. When sodium levels fall below a certain level, which can happen quite fast, there are some undesired side effects such as headaches, low energy, dizziness, and cramping.

> **FUN FACT:** A small fast food milkshake has more sodium in it than fast food french fries, and you wouldn't even know it because of all the sugar.

When you first start your well-formulated low-carb lifestyle, you might notice that if you stand up quickly, you get dizzy or feel faint. This is because you are dehydrated! Just drinking water isn't going to work like it would with a high-carbohydrate diet. You need to add more sodium. You can add more salt to your food, drink bone broth, or take sodium tablets. Salt is not the evil nutrient that your doctor warns you about. You've got to start thinking differently. Just like understanding that eating more fat lowers your risk of heart disease, it is important to understand that a well-formulated low-carb diet requires a more lot more sodium.

My favorite way for clients to get more sodium is to consume homemade bone broth. I have a recipe for this in chapter 9 (Meal Plans and Recipes). This is so easy to make — you can even do it in a slow cooker! Bone broth not only helps with getting sodium, but you also get a ton of minerals and electrolytes. Commercial broth will not have these benefits. It takes a few days to make, but I will often make a huge batch in the pot that Craig used to make home brew in (this was years ago … yes, we have come a long way in our journey). I freeze it in small containers where it keeps for a very long time. Here are some other notes about sodium:

1. Even if you don't have any side effects like edema or headaches, you will need extra water and sodium. Eliminating all packaged foods eliminates a lot of sodium from your diet. As well, the recommended foods

for this diet don't contain a lot of liquid, so you will want to drink at least half your body weight in ounces.

2. If you get the fierce headaches that some people get when starting on a low-carb diet, add sodium. Always drink extra water.

3. If you really don't want to make your own bone broth, you can use store bought bouillon, but please watch for MSG and gluten. Not all brands are healthy. Bouillon has a lot of sodium, tastes really good as a hot drink, and can eliminate carbohydrate cravings.

4. In addition to drinking broth, I suggest you get some Celtic Sea Salt. Himalayan Salt will also work. Throw out your typical store-bought salt and replace it with these natural sea salts. After a few months of using this salt, you will find that if you go to a relative's house or to a restaurant with regular table salt, the salt will have a chemical-like taste.

5. Don't use these Celtic or Himalayan salts sparingly. These salts have either been harvested from ancient sea beds or been made by evaporating seawater with high mineral content and contain about 70% of the sodium of regular salt (which has been refined, bleached, and processed until it is pretty much pure sodium chloride, often with anti-caking agents added). The other 30% is from other minerals and micronutrients (including iodine) found in mineral-rich seas. I greatly prefer these salts taste-wise to regular salt; it is well worth the extra bucks. Do not make the mistake of using Morton Sea Salt, which is devoid of iodine and nutrients.

Potassium

If you don't want to lose lean muscle, pay attention here! Since you lose a lot of sodium through the diuretic effect (loss of water retention) of a low-carb diet, you will eventually lose a lot of potassium as well. Keeping your potassium levels up helps to safeguard your lean muscle mass during weight loss. Also, just as with sodium, adequate potassium levels prevent cramping and fatigue. A deficiency in potassium causes low energy, heavy legs, salt cravings, and dizziness, and you may cry easily. Causes of low potassium would be dehydration from having diarrhea, sweating, and low-carb diets that are not well formulated.

Keeping your sodium as well as your magnesium intake up will help preserve your potassium levels. I often teach nutrition classes, and at the end of each class, I answer questions that participants ask. One question I had was, "How do you recommend getting potassium if you don't recommend eating bananas or potatoes (especially if someone has high blood pressure)?"

I think it is interesting that doctors often recommend bananas and potatoes to their patients when they have high blood pressure. Sure they are going to recommend those things: they taste great, and people love them. But in reality, those two foods are causing the problem, not fixing it! Aside from that, there are foods that are much higher in potassium than the insulin-increasing banana and potato. Dried herbs have a lot more potassium without any of the sugar or starch. And in second place is the avocado!

My Top Choices for Potassium

#1: Dried herbs: Chervil, Parsley, Basil, Dill, Tarragon, Ground Turmeric, Saffron, and Oregano

#2: Avocados

#3: Paprika and red chili powder

#4: Cocoa powder and dark chocolate (especially ChocoPerfection's dark chocolate!)

#5: Nuts: almonds, hazelnuts, pine nuts, coconuts, and walnuts.

#6: Seeds: pumpkin, squash, sunflower, and flax

#7: Fish: pompano, salmon, halibut, and tuna

Let's dive into why eating a banana for the sake of increasing your potassium level is not the greatest idea. Most people who are insulin resistant also have high blood pressure, and insulin resistance is directly caused by a high-sugar, high-grain (even a complex carbs) diet. Complex carbs are just glucose molecules hooked together in long chains; the digestive system then breaks the long chains down into sugar (glucose). So high blood pressure and uncontrolled blood sugar go hand in hand. Insulin also affects your blood pressure by causing your body to retain sodium. Sodium retention causes fluid retention. Fluid retention in turn causes high blood pressure and can lead to congestive heart failure.

To enhance your heart health, the first thing is *not* to remove sodium (though I would get rid of junky table salt and use a quality mineralized salt). You need to remove all grains and sugars, mainly fructose, from your diet until your blood pressure and weight is under control. Eating sugar and grains (including any type of bread, pasta, corn, potatoes, or rice) will cause your insulin levels and your blood pressure to rise.

Fructose is a sugar that can only be metabolized by the liver; it breaks down into a variety of waste products that are unhealthy for your body, one of which is uric acid. Uric acid drives up your blood pressure by inhibiting the nitric oxide in your blood vessels. Nitric oxide helps your vessels maintain their elasticity, so nitric oxide suppression leads to increases in blood pressure. The average American now consumes 70 grams of fructose every day! I will further discuss the damaging effects of fructose in chapter 4 ("The Fat Switch").

> **HEALTH TIP:** There are a couple of prescription medicines that you should be aware of if you significantly increase your potassium intake. If you are on blood pressure medication, talk to your doctor before you take potassium supplements.

To get an adequate amount of potassium, I suggest ingesting about 400 mg a day. You can replenish your potassium by taking 99 mg of potassium supplements four times a day. You can also start adding in some of the foods suggested in the previous list.

Magnesium

A well-formulated keto-adapted diet does not cause a massive depletion of magnesium in your body like a high-carb diet does. For example, your body uses 54 mg of magnesium to process just 1 g of sugar or starch! That creates a high demand for magnesium. No wonder it is one of the most common deficiencies I see in clients. About 70% of people don't even get the minimum recommended daily intake of magnesium, an amount that isn't that high. Most people who have metabolic syndrome, are overweight, insulin resistant, have high blood pressure, or are diabetic are deficient in magnesium. As your insulin level increases, so does your blood pressure. Insulin stores magnesium, but if your insulin receptors are blunted and your cells grow resistant to insulin, you can't store magnesium; therefore, it passes out of your body through urination. Magnesium in your cells relaxes your muscles. If your magnesium level is too low, your blood vessels will constrict rather than relax, which will raise your blood pressure and decrease your energy level.

> **FUN FACT:** Do you suffer from chocolate cravings? This is a sign of a magnesium deficiency. Add in 600-1000 mg of magnesium a day (magnesium glycinate, not oxide) and your cravings will go away!

It is not entirely necessary to get a blood test to see if you are deficient because the fact is that most people don't get enough. Magnesium is a supplement I will always take. It helps repair muscles, naturally relaxes blood vessels and tight muscles, and it is a miracle cure for migraines as well as many other ailments. Good magnesium levels help regulates potassium levels as well. Magnesium is critical for energy production and metabolism, muscle contraction, nerve impulse transmission, and bone mineralization. It is a required cofactor for an estimated three hundred enzymes. Among the reactions catalyzed by these enzymes are fatty acid synthesis, protein synthesis, and glucose metabolism. Magnesium status is also important for regulation of calcium balance through its effects on the parathyroid gland. I suggest supplementing children with this as well, since it helps with sleep issues. Babies can also benefit. There are topical magnesium gels and lotions that are absorbed really well.

> **HEALTH TIP:** We mistakenly blame cholesterol and saturated fats for heart disease, when it is really a magnesium deficiency. Studies have shown that adding 700–1000 mg of magnesium glycinate helps decrease the risk of heart-associated deaths by 70%! I suggest at least 400 mg in the morning when blood pressure is the highest to help naturally relax constricted blood vessels.

You may be wondering why we need to supplement our body with minerals if our ancestors never did. Well, most of the magnesium they ingested was found in the water they drank — now, most people drink treated, softened, or bottled water which are all devoid of magnesium. Magnesium salts in water make deposits in your water pipes, and make it difficult to get a decent lather with soap. This problem was solved with the development of water softeners, but the process gets rid of the magnesium. Our ancestors drank untreated well water or water from a stream which had a lot of magnesium.

Since our water is now depleted, and you don't find adequate amounts of magnesium in foods, I suggest taking a quality chelated magnesium supplement and at least 400 to 1000 mg per day. For most of my clients and their children, magnesium relaxes them, so taking it at bedtime helps them get quality sleep. On rare occasions, magnesium is energizing, so if you find yourself unable to sleep after ingesting magnesium, I suggest taking 400 mg at breakfast and, if needed, another dose at lunch. Everyone has a different tolerance to magnesium. The only problematic side effect is having loose stool. This will happen if you take magnesium oxide that you purchase at a large retail store, which is a non-absorbed form of magnesium. Always look for magnesium glycinate (I have only ever been able to find it online). If you are taking a small dose of magnesium glycinate and still have issues with loose stool, I suggest you use a topical magnesium or Epsom salts in a bath.

> **FUN FACT:** Magnesium is essential for making serotonin. It aids in the conversion of tryptophan, an amino acid, to the neurotransmitter serotonin. A lack of serotonin can lead to depression, insomnia, and migraine headaches.

One of the main symptoms of a magnesium deficiency is hyperactivity and anxiety. A main source of magnesium is "fortified whole grains" (which just means that a magnesium supplement has been added to the grains). So, if you remove gluten from your diet like I suggest you do, you are also removing a major source of magnesium. Since calcium competes with magnesium for uptake, adding in calcium supplements without sufficient magnesium also increases the chance of a magnesium deficiency.

Another thing to note when purchasing magnesium is that chelated magnesium means it is combined with an amino acid agent for absorption. So if the dosage says 1000 mg of magnesium citrate, the amount of magnesium isn't 1000 mg. The chelated amino acid is heavier than magnesium, so about 15% of the weight is magnesium and the rest is the agent. The only way you really know how much magnesium you are getting is to look at the RDI (Recommended Daily Intake). The RDI for magnesium is 400 mg per day. If you see that the dose of the supplement you have contains 50% of the RDI, then you know each dose contains 200 mg of magnesium, regardless of what the dosage is on the front of the bottle.

WATER, WATER, WATER!

Clients often laugh at me when I say you need to drink half of your body weight in ounces, but *not* during meals. When I give them a list of supplements to take at breakfast, they ask, "How am I going to take all of them without drinking?" and "How close to eating can I drink?" and "If I eat every two hours like I am told to do to help 'fuel my metabolism,' when will I have time to drink anything?" Well, first off, if you want to be a fat burner, you cannot eat every two hours! That tip is bogus and unfounded. Sugar burners do need to eat every two hours. You are going to be a fat burner who doesn't need to eat that often. Second, I suggest waking yourself up with a huge glass of water (reverse osmosis water is best). Hydrated cells are energized cells. If you feel tired, sluggish, have a headache, or muscle cramping, ask yourself when the last time you drank water was. Too many clients of mine do not drink enough water. Many times, hunger is simply thirst in disguise.

Drinking half of your body weight in ounces helps out the kidneys and liver. When your kidneys are dehydrated, the liver stops its main jobs and helps out the kidneys. When you are well hydrated, the liver can focus on burning fat. So, be nice to your liver, people!

It is important not to drink during meals because liquids dilute your digestive enzymes. Food breakdown starts in your mouth with chewing and saliva. If you drink a lot while eating, the saliva is washed away. Anyone who suffers from acid reflux or heart burn really needs to stop this habit.

> **HYDRATION TIP:** Coffee, espresso, and tea are diuretics that will cause cramping and dehydration. Alcohol is also a diuretic, but you're not going to drink alcohol anyway, right!? If you think that drinking a pot of coffee a day counts towards your liquid intakes, think again.

Hydration has a lipolytic, or fat-burning, effect. Research clearly demonstrates that dieters who consume a lot of water have increased lipolysis. When you drink water, especially ice-cold water, your body burns calories in order to bring the water to body temperature, but that increase doesn't amount to all that much. Your blood also dilutes for a bit until the water equilibrates with the fluid in all the tissues, an effect that takes some time. When the blood is diluted, the amount of various substances traveling in the bloodstream decreases, which means that insulin levels fall. Blood volume is about 5 L. If you drink a liter of water, this will momentarily increase the blood volume by about 20%, and therefore cause the concentration of insulin and other molecules in the blood to fall by 20%. A 20% drop in insulin levels allows fat to release from the fat cells and enables transit into the mitochondria for burning.

> **FUN FACT:** Don't get sucked into the goofy fads like "seaweed body wrapping" to help you lose inches. They just suck all the water out of your cells and create a dehydrated effect. As you just read, hydration = fat burning!

Hydration is important to pay attention to when starting off a keto-adapted low-carb diet because excess ketones are released through the kidneys along with a lot of liquid. This is one reason why "low-carbers" will complain of headaches and low energy at first: their diet isn't a "well-formulated" program. You need to intentionally increase your liquids to at least half your body weight in ounces, and increase your sodium intake as well. You should be taking more than that at first, but once you are well into your keto-adapted state, you should aim for that amount.

> **HEALTH TIP:** Reverse osmosis water is devoid of minerals. I suggest re-mineralizing the water by adding a pinch of Celtic Sea Salt to each of your bottles (just enough so it doesn't taste too salty).

I find that clients have the most success with hydration when they have a plan. In the morning, fill your glass water bottles with reverse osmosis water. If you aren't a fan of plain water, I suggest getting a soda streamer and adding tasty stevia drops. My husband and I love fruit punch stevia in fizzy water. When you get into a routine of drinking a certain amount of ounces right away when you wake up, and then another goal amount between each meal, you get into a habit. Do something sixteen times in a row and it becomes a habit. Consider today day one of your new hydration habit. Get those glass water bottles ready!

I get asked a lot about coffee. I'm not totally against it unless you have adrenal fatigue or a thyroid issue. The main thing to think about is that coffee is a very heavy, pesticide-sprayed product. Choose organic first. Decaf coffee usually tastes terrible, so what I do is I make a decaf Americano, which tastes amazing! An Americano is a shot of espresso with hot water added to it. Espresso in general has less caffeine than coffee does — making it decaf ensures that you don't dehydrate your cells further.

I also get asked why I do not recommend alcohol. I wrote a whole sub-chapter on alcohol in my book *Secrets to a Healthy Metabolism*, so I won't bore you here with the depressing details of that. But I would like to summarize a few points:

1. Fat metabolism is reduced by around 73% after only two alcoholic beverages in a one-hour time period. This scary fact shows that the worst thing about alcohol is not so much how many calories it contains, but how it stops your body from using your fat stores for energy.

2. When alcohol is consumed, the body converts it into a substance called acetate. Studies find that blood levels of acetate are 2.5 times higher than normal after only two drinks. This quick rise in blood acetate puts the brakes on fat burning.

3. The more you drink, the more you tend to eat. Unfortunately, drinking will make your liver work to convert the alcohol into acetate, which means that the foods you consume at this time will be converted into extra fat on your body.

4. Alcohol decreases your testosterone levels for up to 24 hours after you finish drinking. Athletes make a huge mistake by lifting weights the morning before a night of drinking in order to "earn their calories." As you lift weights, you break down your muscle; as you rest, you rebuild muscle and get more muscle ... but you need testosterone in order for

this to happen. Therefore, if you work out really hard Friday morning and binge drink Friday night, you will wake up on Saturday morning with a slower metabolism than you had on Friday! Alcohol causes a quicker aromatization of androgens into estrogens, which explains why men who are heavy drinkers often get gynecomastia (enlarged breasts) over a period of time. A "beer belly" isn't really a beer belly, it is an "estrogen belly!"

5. We all know that alcohol dehydrates us. In order for fat to be metabolized, it must first be released from the fat cell and then be transported by the bloodstream, where it is pushed to the liver to be used as fuel. If you are dehydrated, the liver has to come to the aid of the kidneys and can't focus on its role of releasing fat.

Is that enough reason to skip that glass of wine at night? If not, one more fact: grapes are one of the most pesticide-sprayed fruits. Where does wine come from? Grapes, and it is very concentrated. So when you drink wine, you are ingesting a lot of pesticides, too.

Checking your Ketones

There are two ways to check your ketones at home: you can use urine test strips or blood test strips. Below is a summary of each of these methods for checking your keto adaption.

Urine Strips

Urine strips are less expensive and can give you a rough idea of what state you are in. The testing strip will display a varying shade of color and depending on how dark, a range of ketones that corresponds to. They typically have six color ranges that go from little or no ketones (very little color) up to very high ketone levels (very dark color). Urine strips are pretty inaccurate, however, so I suggest using the blood tester (unless you are diabetic and need to check everyday for ketoacidosis or if cost is a concern).

Blood Tester

The blood test strips are just like glucose test strips. In fact, the ketone tester my husband and I use (Nova Max Plus) also does glucose levels. The blood test strips are much more accurate than the urine strips, and you get a numerical readout of your ketone level, too, which is useful. The drawback is that the test strips are very expensive (about $2 each). I suggest using these as a spot check to determine when you have reached ketosis (so you know what level of fat, protein, and carbs will get you there) and then spot check when you try new foods as change your ratios.

Ketosis is defined as 0.5 to 5.0 mmol. Ideally you want to have about 2 mmol for optimum weight loss and healing. If you reach 10–15 mmol, seek a doctor, as this is ketoacidosis and can be life threatening (though this typically occurs only in extreme type 1 diabetics who haven't managed their insulin levels).

Here is another testimony from a client becoming keto-adapted:

"I just wanted to send my thank yous. I have been following you for a while, have all of your cookbooks and love your recipes. Recently (the last two months), my weight loss stalled. I've lost 70 lbs since last year and have another 50 to go (down 110 lbs from my heaviest weight). My husband has lost 75 lbs. I was keeping my carbs under 30g but didn't pay any attention to my protein and fat.

1 1/2 weeks ago, I started tracking everything. 5% carbs, 15% protein and 80% fat. Although my fat intake isn't quite there, I (counter-intuitively) upped my fat dramatically. Lo and behold, I'm losing again!

I work, I go to school full-time (graduating in December...wahoo!!!), I'm a wife, mom and grandma. Life is super busy but I make sure to make the time to cook. I spend Saturday mornings baking. Through Maria, and further study, I have become very aware of what is in food and make my choices accordingly. Please, don't ever feel defeated. I didn't think I could do this but I did. I've heard it from others...If I can do this, so can you! This is now our lifestyle. This is not a "diet". We will be eating like this for the rest of our lives. We're losing weight, our blood pressure is down, we're getting off of medication...and we're looking good too! I just want to say thank you to Maria again! She's made this transformation "easy" through her writings, her explanations (it's easier to make choices when it makes sense and Maria is great helping it make sense) and all of her wonderful recipes!

On a side note, we also have a 14 year old son. In the last year of making these changes, he has only lost 5 lbs (he was pretty heavy as well)...however, he grew 5 inches. He went from 5'7" and 195 lbs to 6'0" and 190 lbs. He's looking fantastic! Very proud of him as well.

I've spent decades overweight, following a 1200 calorie diet, low fat and whole grains. Amazing that now I'm eating almost 2000 calories, low carb/high fat diet, I'm still shedding the weight! Thank you for all of your advice! This has been an amazing transformation of my life!"

—*Maryann*

Summary:

Becoming keto-adapted can change your health for the better in ways you never imagined possible. This lifestyle will improve your long term health and quality of life. It may seem like a very limited style of eating, but with my passion for cooking, I have created many recipes that are keto and will help you stay on track while enjoying tasty food. Don't wait another day; start experiencing the benefits now!

Chapter 3

Health Benefits of Being Keto-Adapted

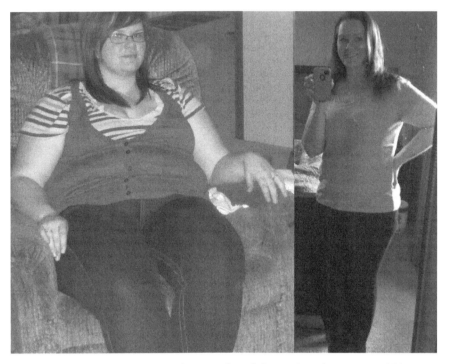

Hi, Maria! I'm Alexis. I am a military wife and the mother of a six-year-old boy and a three-year-old girl. My husband is deployed right now. This [problem] all started after Christmas of 2010.

I was horrified to see a picture of myself during the holidays looking like a blob. This particular holiday, I had put on at least 10 lbs (10 LBS!) over the course of two weeks. I had told myself after having my daughter the year before, and even after having my son in '08 (I was 301 lbs when I went into the hospital to have him), that I was going to be what I should be, what I deserve to be, for the children, for my husband, and for myself. Everything ended up being a constant struggle of starvation and binge eating, all of which was getting me nowhere fast. I've always been huge. I can remember at the beginning of middle school tipping the scales at 200 lbs. But that picture was it for me. No more.

I started out with Weight Watchers. People lose weight on this program, right? I was losing some weight, but just not as quickly as I had hoped to. I came across a company *that has some pretty great products with people having amazing results! After seeing what the distributors of these items were telling people to eat, it appeared to me that people were starving themselves to get the results so quickly. I still bought into the company, but applied my own ways of eating. I ate healthy whole grains with lots of fruits and veggies, along with all fat-free items! That year I lost 50 lbs in eight months. Not bad, right? But I always craved, always longed for cake, chocolate, and potato chips! I fell right back into my old patterns and put on 30 lbs. :(*

I had pains. Carpel tunnel mostly. I swore my bed was made out of rocks and cursed the day I bought the stupid thing. I woke up every morning feeling like I had been beaten. Then came (what I swear was gall bladder pain) acid reflex, It just wasn't coming up, it was sitting there burning in my stomach area. Oh, I called it the "great pain" … for hours I would sit and cry. Sometimes it would bring me to the point of vomiting. I was prescribed one of those pain-go-away-quickly meds. It worked, but I hated being on meds for the pain.

You are so inspiring. The first book I purchased was The Art of Healthy Eating - Kids *cookbook. [My kids] are the ones I really want to help from falling into these vicious ways. I just recently bought the* Healthy Metabolism *book which I am so excited about! I'm reading away. But just by doing the little bit that I have, I'm down to 215 lbs at the moment. Started out around 280 lbs in Feb. 2011, and was around 250 lbs in March of this year (2013). My arm pains are still diminishing. I love my bed now and cannot wait to sleep in it. Oh, and the "great pain" is gone, no meds. I know I'm just beginning my journey and my family's journey. I do have a long way to go. There are more bad habits I need to drop and healthy ones to gain (e.g. more exercise), but I thought I would share my progress with you. Thank you!*

—*Alexis*

BENEFIT #1: Brain Health and Mitochondria Energy

A ketogenic diet isn't something that has been recently formulated. People have been on ketogenic diets for virtually three million years, during which time our brains grew and evolved. Now, not only is the human brain shrinking, but brain atrophy has become the norm as we age. We are plagued with diseases such as dementia, Alzheimer's disease, and Parkinson's disease.

Our brain, organs, and tissues work much better when they use ketones as a source of fuel. The heart and the brain work at least 25% more efficiently on ketones than they do on glucose. Ketones are the ideal fuel for our bodies, unlike glucose, which is damaging, less stable, more excitatory, and in fact, shortens your life span. There is something called glycation, where glucose binds to proteins (more on this in chapter 4). This process produces free radicals and inflammation, which are markers of Alzheimer's. It is quite easy to do a test and see if you have this happening in your body. If your Hemoglobin A1c is high, it increases free radicals by fifty-fold. Studies show that this is a marker for the progression of atrophy of the brain.[6] Ketones aren't just fuel for our body, but they are also great for our brain. They provide substrates to help repair damaged neurons and membranes. This is why I really push a high-fat and low-carb diet for clients who suffer from Alzheimer's (sometimes referred to as type 3 diabetes) and seizures.

Ketones are non-glycating, which is to say that they don't have a caramelizing aging effect on your body. The mitochondria are the "powerhouse" energy-producing factories of our cells. They work much better on a ketogenic diet because they can increase energy levels in an unwavering, long lasting, and efficient way.

A ketogenic diet also increases the energetic output of our mitochondria because these amazing "powerhouse" factories of our cells are essentially designed to use fat as energy. When we switch from using glucose to using fat in the mitochondria, its toxic burden is reduced, the manifestation of energy-producing genes are improved, the output is increased, and the load of inflammatory by-products is decreased.

Glucose needs to be processed first in the cell before it can be passed into the "powerhouse" factory mitochondria. Energy sources from fat don't need this processing: they go straight into the mitochondria for energy. It is more intricate to create energy out of glucose than out of fat, which causes you to get more energy per molecule of fat than glucose. I see so many clients with fibromyalgia, chronic fatigue, rheumatoid arthritis, cancer, multiple sclerosis, and other autoimmune diseases that cause energy shortages. The ketogenic diet acts on numerous levels at once, something that no drug has been able to do without detrimental side effects.

It's quite possible you are skimming over this information, bored out of your mind. I certainly did the same thing in my biology class when I was in high school. But not only is this science simple, it can actually be quite fascinating. Think of the mitochondria as the main sources of energy for your cells and body. The energy produced by mitochondria is stored in a molecule called adenosine triphosphate (ATP) — you can consider this your body's "battery." Energy-packed ATP can then be transported throughout the cell, releasing energy on-demand of specific enzymes. In addition to the fuel they produce, mitochondria also create a by-product related to oxygen called reactive oxygen species (ROS), commonly known as free radicals. But free radicals are not produced if we use fat for fuel instead of carbohydrates.

In some cells, mitochondria compose 50% of the total volume! When we are low in energy and need a boost, true energy doesn't come from a short-lived sugar boost from carbohydrates. That energy does not last long and is not without its consequences; it is sort of like how drinking coffee gives us false energy. Instead, true long-term energy comes from the mitochondria. I once read, "Let fat be thy medicine and medicine be thy fat!" How true!

MYTH #1: We need glucose for brain function

According to certain health authorities, the recommended daily minimum for carbohydrates is 130 grams. The reason for this is that the brain is assumed to be dependent on glucose for fuel. This is half true. There are certain neurons in the brain that can't burn anything but glucose, but other parts of the brain prefer ketone bodies. When we eat very little carbohydrates, our requirement for glucose goes down. Some parts of the brain start burning ketone bodies instead of glucose. Even when we eat zero carbohydrates, the body can produce the glucose it needs from protein through a process known as gluconeogenesis.[7]

Keto-adapted diets don't starve the brain, and they don't make you feel slow in the beginning when you are not yet keto-adapted. Give it time, and you will have more energy than you ever thought possible.

BENEFIT #2: Decrease in Risk of Coronary Artery Disease

Photo: The meal my father-in-law was served after his stroke in August 2013!

The following is a testimonial of a client and her improvements eliminating sugar and grains:

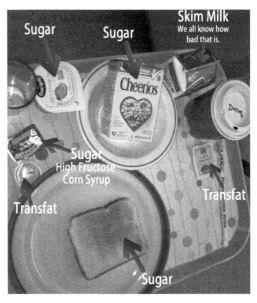

I have to tell you about a recent doctor visit. I told my doc that I'd started working with a nutritionist (you) and changed my diet rather dramatically. He asked a bunch of questions about it. I told him that I completely eliminated both sugar and grains. He seemed really pleased about that and kept asking questions. I told him that he may be horrified by this, but I added way *more fat into my diet. He said that he wasn't horrified at all and was really pleased to hear it. Then he looked through my chart and told me that I'd lost about 13 pounds since the last time I'd been in (maybe a year ago). We decided it would be good to get some blood work done at this time, just to see how I compare to my last blood work-up.*

He left a rather long-winded message on my cell phone last night, and suffice it to say, he was waxing lyrical about my results. He said they were really, really great all around. Even my thyroid labs, which had been a problem in the past. He ended the diatribe by saying that with regards to my cholesterol, he joked that he was going to hang the results on the wall to let everyone gawk at. Haha!

—MJ

My grandpa Vince survived his first heart attack at age 32, but with the diet that his doctor recommended, it is no wonder his heart never healed. He eventually required heart surgery at age 45, and then another one at age 52. At that point, the doctors gave him five years to live; he made it to nine and died at age 61. He was given nutrition advice from his doctor to never eat eggs, butter, or saturated fat. He was living off of fake butter substitutes and popcorn. There were other factors that increased his risk of heart disease: He owned a business which was very stressful. I also remember him smoking a pipe. My dad mentioned to me the other day that with the knowledge we now have, and with the aid of my recipes, he knows Grandpa Vince would have lived a lot longer.

> **HEALTH TIP:** Our brain is over 25% cholesterol. A deficiency can lead to Alzheimer's.[24]

Cholesterol is not the bad guy that we have vilified; it is vital for every cell in your body. You cannot live one day without it! It does not damage arteries, but actually repairs arteries.[8] I like to refer to cholesterol as the firefighters in our body. They help fight the inflammation that is occurring. Sure, your cholesterol numbers will go down if you kill the firefighters, but did the inflammation (the fire) go away? No, it didn't.

Cholesterol is so important to the human body that nature has devised a backup plan in the event that your diet falls short. When that happens, your liver steps in to make cholesterol to give your body a baseline level. The high levels of insulin that are released in a low-fat, high-carb diet trigger the body to tap off leftover blood sugar into the liver, making cholesterol and triglycerides, which are used for energy and fat storage.

In its natural, unstressed state, your liver makes 75% of the cholesterol your body needs. The rest you have to eat (this includes my favorite group of foods): butter, meat, whole-fat dairy products, shellfish, and eggs.

If you deprive yourself of cholesterol, your liver will overproduce it to make up the difference. This overdrive state can't shut off until you start eating cholesterol again. So, a low-cholesterol, high-carbohydrate diet can actually lead to heart disease.

> **HEALTH TIP:** When you get your cholesterol levels checked, wait six months after your weight has stabilized. When you eat a keto-adapted diet, you lose weight by burning body fat rather than lean mass, like you do with low-fat diets. For example, if you are losing one pound of body fat every four days, that is 3500 calories worth of animal fat that goes into your blood as triglycerides. If you get your blood drawn in the middle of your well-formulated, keto-adapted weight loss journey, there's a good chance that your numbers will look "bad" to your doctor. Triglycerides may be very high since your blood is now full of them because they are getting released from your fat cells.

The biggest contributor to heart disease risk is inflammation. A well-formulated keto-adapted diet produces very little inflammation. Sugar and carbs are the big culprits when it comes to increased inflammation. Coronary artery disease occurs when a low-density lipoprotein particle (LDL) gets lodged into a lesion (caused by inflammation) in the artery wall. This particle then releases its cholesterol into the artery wall which starts the formation of plaque. So if you have very low inflammation and no arterial lesions for the LDL to get stuck in, your cholesterol numbers aren't really relevant. Dr. Dwight Lundell summarizes this conclusion in the following statements: "We've long known that atherosclerosis is an inflammatory disease. In the absence of inflammation or injury to the endothelial cell, the cholesterol would never go through the arterial wall and it would never stay there."[59]

Given this, the much better markers for coronary artery risk are your inflammation markers: post-meal blood sugar levels, C-reactive protein (CRP), and your Triglyceride (TG) to HDL ratio. You want a fasting blood sugar level that is below 90, and a postprandial level below 140. CRP levels should be less than 1.0, and your TG/HDL ratio less than 2 (ideally less than 1).

HEALTH TIP: "The Triglyceride-to-HDL ratio should not be used in African-Americans. They just don't have high triglycerides, even if they have severe insulin resistance. Why? Because they have different types of lipase, the enzyme that catabolize triglyceride expression. African-Americans' insulin resistance is better characterized by glucose abnormalities, obesity and high blood pressure, not high triglycerides and low HDL cholesterol." [59] - Dr. Thomas Dayspring

The following quotation is from Dr. Stephanie Seneff who is a senior scientist at MIT and has been conducting research for over three decades:

Heart disease, I think, is a cholesterol deficiency problem, and in particular a cholesterol sulfate deficiency problem ... The macrophages in the plaque take up LDL, the small dense LDL particles that have been damaged by sugar ... The liver cannot take them back because the receptor can't receive them, because they are gummed with sugar basically. So they're stuck floating in your body ... Those macrophages in the plaque do a heroic job in taking that gummed up LDL out of the blood circulation, carefully extracting the cholesterol from it to save it – the cholesterol is important – and then exporting the cholesterol into HDL – HDL A1 in particular ... That's the good guy, HDL. The platelets in the plaque take in HDL A1 cholesterol and they won't take anything else ... They take in sulfate, and they produce cholesterol sulfate in the plaque. The sulfate actually comes from homocysteine. Elevated homocysteine is another risk factor for heart disease. Homocysteine is a source of sulfate. It also involves hemoglobin. You have to consume energy to produce a sulfate from homocysteine, and the red blood cells actually supply the ATP to the plaque.

So everything is there and the intent is to produce cholesterol sulfate and it's done in the arteries feeding the heart, because it's the heart that needs the cholesterol sulfate. If [cholesterol sulfate is not produced] ... you end up with heart failure.[9]

To increase sulfur in your diet, add fresh garlic and onions to food daily. Beware, though: cooking onions for even ten minutes destroys sulfates. Keep in mind as well that you need adequate amounts of sunlight to be able to absorb sulfur.

Let's review! Well-formulated keto-adapted diets:

1. Reduce body fat much more than low-fat diets, even though the low-carb groups are allowed to eat until fullness.[10, 11]
2. Lower blood sugar and improve symptoms of diabetes.[12]
3. Increase HDL cholesterol (the good kind) much more than low-fat diets.[13]
4. Change the pattern of LDL cholesterol (the bad kind) from small, dense LDL (the very bad kind) to large LDL.[14, 15]
5. Cause a greater reduction in blood pressure.[16, 17]
6. Lower blood triglycerides.[18]

In conclusion, well-formulated keto-adapted diets improve *all* biomarkers of health to a much greater extent than the low-fat diets still recommended by the authorities.

The following is a testimonial from a client who is on track to heart health:

I have been meaning to send you a quick note and let you know of our continued efforts with this journey to be "healthified."... And there's nothing to spur me on like people talking smack to my girl! I just want to remind you how awesome you are, how much you have helped us, and how you are continuing to change peoples lives! Thank you, Maria, for sharing your God-given talent with the world! You have changed our lives ... without finding you 2 1/2 years ago, my feeble attempts at eating low-carb would have come to a halt. One can only eat so much meat and pork rinds before you get really, really tired of it.

You have opened our world up to a whole new way of eating without feeling deprived. Thank you!

(Same sender, new email)

So after feeling defeated my husband went and had his blood work done and here are his results: his A1c went from 6.2 to 5.7. Yay! His TC went from 190 to 162 ... HDL 53 to 48 ... Trg 91 to 78 ... LDL 119 to 98 ... Non HDL 138 to 114 ... TC/HDL 3.6 to 3.4. This is without meds; he quit taking those almost a year ago. This report thoroughly convinced him to eat "Maria's way" 100% of the time.

As for me, well, I have found a doctor who is working with me to try to get my hormones balanced. I go back mid-July to discuss the results of the blood work, saliva and stool test. After my first visit, the doctor put me on Livothyronine Sodium tablets ... my thyroid is a little sluggish! But if it weren't for you, I would have accepted what the other doctors had advised and not have ever known that I have a allergy to dairy and a slow thyroid. I would probably be on a anti-depressant for menopausal symptoms, too. You continue to motivate me. Now, at almost 54 years-old, I am doing a body pump class. At 53, I ran two 5ks (never liked running before) and feel better than I did 15-20 years ago! You are changing lives and lifestyles. Thank- you! I will give you an update in July after I hear what the doctor says. I would still love for the number on the scales to go down ... that for me is a never-ending struggle. But unlike in previous years, it's not going up either. Yay! One small victory!

Be blessed, and know that you have many, many people all around the world who love you and care about you (and your family) and thank God for you everyday.

Oh, and just a side note: I walk/jog three miles in the morning, ride my bike two miles, walk in the evening, body pump twice a week, clean houses five days a week, have a garden, and mow the yard with a push mower instead of using the rider (just so I get my exercise). I only wish all my efforts would work like they did for you!

— Beverly

> **HEALTH TIP:** Higher thyroid numbers cause higher cholesterol because they interfere with how effectively your liver breaks down and excretes cholesterol in the bile. So high cholesterol is a suggestion to get your thyroid checked.

There is one fat that you should toss from your pantry and it lurks in just about every prepackaged food item: anything with the words "partially hydrogenated oil" has to go. One reason why trans-fats are so bad is that they interfere with our cells' ability to metabolize omega-3 fats. Trans-fats damage cell membranes of vital structures of our brain and nerve cells. With all the information we have out there about the dangers of trans-fats, I almost cut this information out of this book, but we obviously need to keep preaching about it. Serving margarine to a pregnant woman should be criminal!

The following is from a client and talk about their experience with hospital food:

When I was pregnant with my first child twelve years ago, I was diagnosed with gestational diabetes. That didn't surprise me as both my mother and sister are diabetics. I was sent to the diabetic nurse and hospital nutritionist for 'diet' changes. What they didn't know is that I was already following a modified Atkins diet because of my family history. This is where I realized that the so called diabetic diet that they were teaching their patients was hopelessly flawed. They asked me to write down everything I ate, so I did. It consisted mostly of eggs, red meat, fresh low-glycemic veggies, almond milk, etc. Basically no sugar or wheat of any kind because I knew it would raise my blood sugar which was unhealthy for my baby. Boy oh boy, did I get a blast from both the nurse and the nutritionist. They were horrified that I was consuming less than 100 carbs a day! They said that is why we have insulin to regulate your blood sugar; you need carbohydrates to grow a healthy baby. What a load of crock! So from then on, forgive [me] for saying [it], but I lied every week on my diet journal so that they wouldn't give me any flack. The outcome: two very healthy baby boys. Yes, I did the process all over again for my second pregnancy. Oh, and when I was in the hospital giving birth, do you know what they fed me afterwards? Macaroni and cheese, 2% milk, jello, green peas and a bun with bagel margarine. Yikes! I didn't touch it, my husband snuck food in for me.

—*Cindy from Canada*

> **HEALTH TIP:** In a tiny percent of people, there is a disorder called familial hypercholesterolemia, where they have radically high levels of low-density lipoprotein cholesterol (LDL), which can lead to accelerated atherosclerosis. It is a genetic disorder caused by a defect on chromosome 19. The reason why someone may want to get tested for this disorder is because if they pro-create with someone who also has this genetic disorder, the baby often dies at a very young age.

Imagine this: we have "parking spots" that are specifically designed to receive certain molecules. When omega-3s "park," they fill assigned parking spots and contribute to the health of the membrane. However, if trans-fatty acid "cars" come along, they try to squeeze into a space that doesn't fit. A biochemical traffic jam occurs, and the right cars can't get to where they need to be.

Two problems occur in this "jam": First, the molecular misfit "car" is left to wander throughout the body, causing damage in other places. Second, these misfit "cars" keep pushing their way in, damaging themselves and the "cars" around them. The damage caused by these misfits also changes the shape of the cellular membrane, causing the right "cars" (the healthy nutrients) to no longer fit.

Hydrogenated fats can weaken cell membranes, keeping out needed nutrients and also allowing harmful ones to leak in. This causes inflammation, which will increase cholesterol, but cholesterol isn't the bad guy. Remember, cholesterol acts as the firefighters that are trying to put out the fire (inflammation). We need to heal inflammation, *not* take a prescription drug that kills the firefighters. Put out the fire, not the firefighters!

Hydrogenated fats, found in margarine and Jiff peanut butter, interfere with the absorption of the anti-inflammatory omega-3 fats. Good omega-3 fats open receptors, but hydrogenated fats basically form a crust around cells and block glucose from entering. This forces the glucose to float around in the bloodstream where it turns into triglycerides. This is why diabetics have high rates of heart disease.

MYTH #2: YOU NEED TO EAT EVERY 2 TO 3 HOURS TO "FUEL YOUR METABOLISM" AND "BREAKFAST IS THE MOST IMPORTANT MEAL OF THE DAY"

One question frequently pops up from clients: "I'm not hungry for lunch, but I'm afraid I shouldn't skip it because it will slow my metabolism. Should I eat anyway?" Absolutely not! We must stop believing that we "need" 5 to 6 small meals per day to fire up that metabolism and keep a stable blood sugar. If we are constantly filling our bodies with food, the hormone insulin rises. Insulin is an antagonist to the human growth hormone (or HGH, our fat-burning hormone) and will lead to weight gain, not loss. Instead, adopt the Grandma Diet, also called the no "S" diet, which is no Sweets, no Snacks, no Seconds, except on Special events.

The studies that indicate eating multiple small meals will increase your metabolism are very misleading. The energy output of eating, also called the "thermogenic effect," is so insignificant (unless you are a bodybuilder) and it is irrelevant in most circumstances.[19] On the contrary, studies on intermittent fasting have showed that extended periods without eating can be outstanding for your metabolism because it creates an improved hormone regulation of leptin and ghrelin, among other benefits.[20] More importantly, the studies show that it's way more important what you eat than when you eat it.

As soon as you eat breakfast, you "break your fat-burning fast." Contrary to what those popular diet magazines suggest, do not eat right away when you wake up. Breakfast is not the most important meal of the day: your first meal of the day is the most important. I wake up at 5 a.m. to do some work until about 8 a.m., run from 8 a.m. to 9 a.m., and then I eat. I have never been more fit and muscular in my life.

BENEFIT #3: A Keto-Adapted Diet Stops Feeding Cancer Cells

On February 15th, 2013, I was diagnosed with a 12mm pineal gland cyst after a sever migraine. In late July, I flew to Colorado in the hopes of finding some answers and second opinions. I was given no information from the 2-3 neurologists that I have seen as to what caused or what is "feeding" this. The doctors are very unhelpful due to where my cyst is located (dead center of my brain). They're fearful that it will grow (thus forcing them to operate), so they shove RXs at me in the hopes that something will help. Only more bad news followed. Not only was the cyst causing problems, I was on my way to getting type 2 diabetes and leaky gut. I knew I needed to change my life and fast.

I found out about "the Maria Way" from some very good friends. I have followed your plan since the beginning of August. On August 20th, 2013, just two and a half short weeks of being GF, I had my follow up MRI. It showed that the cyst was now only 1.1 cm in size. It had already shrunk 1 mm! I know that sounds tiny but when you're talking about something growing in the middle of your brain it means a lot! I have stopped all meds and have been migraine- and headache-free for almost a month now, thanks to you!

My skin has also improved and my body has never felt better. I can't wait to see how I feel in a month! My holistic doctors believe that a change in diet and taking the right supplements will probably shrink or even make my cyst go away. I am really looking forward to total body health. I truly do feel that "you are what you eat."

I have never felt better. Not only am I losing weight, but very soon I will be completely healthy. Thank you, Maria!

—Megan

Why are the rates of cancer going up? In 1840, the average American consumed 2 teaspoons of sugar a day … in 2011, the typical American consumes over 63 teaspoons of sugar per day! Cancer *loves* glucose. This is why we test cancer patients by having them drink a "glucose mix" and watch which cells consume the glucose the quickest (the answer is cancer cells). So you might think, "Sure, let's just cut out the glucose from our diet." Most people, however, don't understand where all the glucose is coming from. It isn't just the sugar. As I have discussed in earlier chapters, our bodies break down complex carbohydrates into glucose; so, a sugary diet and a starchy diet are pretty much the same thing. In essence, a bowl of oatmeal with skim milk and a banana is just a huge bowl of sugar. For about five years now, German doctors have been testing cancer patients in a clinical study of a surprising prescription … fat. Their patients are on a ketogenic diet, which eliminates almost all carbohydrates and sugar, and provides energy only from high-quality fats.

A well-formulated ketogenic diet has an intense and fast effect on cancer. All of your body's cells, including cancer cells, are fueled by glucose. Conversely, cancer cells have one huge mortal flaw: they do not have the metabolic adaptability to be fueled by ketones, but your healthy cells can thrive on ketones. Therefore, since cancer cells need glucose to thrive, and carbohydrates turn into glucose in your body, then cutting out carbs literally starves the cancer cells.

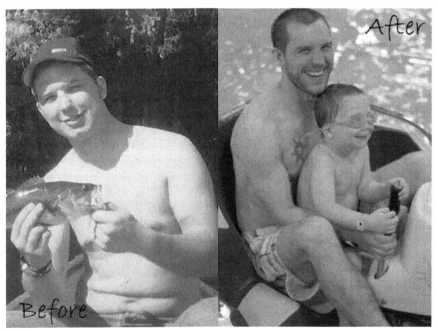

My story begins with my three-year-old son and his journey through cancer. Our family had already discovered the "Maria Way" a few years ago, but we had not fully put it into practice. A little over a year ago, tragedy hit when we

discovered our little three-year-old boy had a five-pound cancerous tumor at-tached to his kidney. After major surgery and a five day hospital stay, we knew we needed to change our nutrition. If there were ever a time for taking drastic measure it was then. We consulted with Maria and cleaned out every ounce of sugar and grains from our house.

Our young family of four all adopted a new way of eating, a new way of life. Since I have such a loving committed wife who took care of most of the cooking, you could say I was more or less along for the ride. I was surprised to find that this journey had many unexpected benefits right from the start.

When we began eating the "Maria Way," I weighed in at over 200 pounds. Just a few months later I had lost just over 40 pounds. I have had multiple knee surgeries and suffer from arthritis and joint pain, however since we kicked the grains and sugar I have little to no soreness ever. Stairs were an issue, but no longer are. I sleep through night regularly now, and my energy level is through the roof. You could say the kids also had this same benefit!

Though this way of eating (menu planning/prep work/etc.) can be difficult at times, it has brought our family together in love and in the kitchen! Our son has been doing fantastic with perfect check ups. Our family has been learning about new foods and how to be betters cooks and could not have done it without Maria's help.

—Joe

Now you may be thinking, "This sounds like the complete opposite of the 'raw food' juicing cancer diets that I have been reading about!" But the scientific evidence for these facts dates back more than eighty years. In 1924, Nobel Prize–winner Otto Warburg published his observations of a common feature he saw in fast-growing tumors: unlike healthy cells that can get energy by metabolizing fat in the mitochondria (ketosis), cancer cells appeared to fuel themselves only through glycolysis, a less efficient means of creating energy through the fermentation of sugar in the cyto-plasm. Warburg believed that this metabolic switch was the primary cause of cancer, a theory that he was unable to prove before his death.

If most aggressive cancers rely on the fermentation of sugar for growing and dividing, then removing sugar from your diet can stop the spread of cancer. Now that sugar has been taken away,, normal body and brain cells make the switch to using fatty ketone molecules to generate energy, the body's main source of energy on a fat-rich diet.

One inaccurate theory that has unfortunately stuck with cancer patients is that diet can influence our body's pH balance (level of acidity). This concept is known as the acid-alkaline theory. This theory has generated a number of books that wrongly encourage these alkaline diets for preventing and curing cancer. In reality, cancer cells are a bit more acidic just outside their boundaries than inside due to the expelling of lactic acid. It seems that trying to control the level of acidity in your body has no real affect on the cancer cells. Not only does the absence of acid in the gastric tract and bladder establish an environment that is favorable to tumor growth, but the control of pH is automatically controlled in a neutral range of 7.2–7.4. Our diets have been proven to have little to no effect over the pH of the blood.

> **HEALTH TIP:** Excess "bad" estrogen in the liver and fat cells is a leading cause of breast, thyroid, and uterine cancer in women and prostate cancer in men. Cutting out all of the estrogenic factors listed in the menopause section of this book is extremely important. A supplement called EstroFactors helps detox this bad estrogen out of the liver, which will in turn heal liver function and increase T3 production for thyroid patients.

A ketogenic diet is helpful for cancer patients for many reasons. For one, it decreases the buildup of lactate, which helps control pH and respiratory function. A myth of low-carb diets is that it puts you in a state of ketoacidosis. Dr. Volek and Phinney write in *The Art and Science of Low Carbohydrate Living*, "This stems from the unfortunate fact that many doctors confuse nutritional ketosis (blood ketones at 1-3 millimolar) with keto-acidosis (blood ketones greater than 15 millimolar). In nutritional ketosis, blood pH at rest stays normal, plus sharp drops in pH due to CO_2 and lactate buildup during exercise are restrained. By contrast, in keto-acidosis, blood pH is driven abnormally low by the 10-fold greater buildup of ketones. Suggesting these 2 states are similar is like equating a gentle rain with a flood because they both involve water."

> **HEALTH TIP:** Do you complain of sagging skin or cellulite? A high-carbohydrate diet causes a natural process called glycation, where the sugar in your bloodstream attaches to proteins to form harmful new molecules called advanced glycation end-products, or AGEs. The more carbohydrates you eat, the more AGEs you develop. As AGEs accumulate, they damage neighboring proteins in a domino-like manner. Collagen and elastin are the protein fibers that keep skin firm and elastic and are most vulnerable when you are eating a high starch diet. Once the damage has been done, the supple and strong collagen and elastin become dry and delicate, leading to wrinkles and sagging. AGEs deactivate your body's natural antioxidant enzymes, leaving you more vulnerable to sun damage. Adding in 600 mg of alpha-lipoic acid (ALA) can help repair the skin from your past years of being a sugar burner. If you are going to spend the money on ALA supplements and serums, make sure to get it from a quality source from Germany. Chinese ALA is processed with harsh and toxic chemicals.

A ketogenic diet doesn't damage our immune system like a high-carb diet does and it has less free radical damage in our cells. Free radicals are highly reactive molecules produced in the mitochondria that damage protein tissues and membranes of the cells. Free radicals are generated as we exercise. Ketones, on the other hand, are a "clean-burning fuel." When ketones are the fuel source, the ROS level (number of oxygen-free radicals) is drastically reduced. Intense exercise on a high-carb diet overwhelms the antioxidant defenses and cell membranes, which explains why extreme athletes have impaired immune systems and decreased gut (intestinal) health. A well-designed ketogenic diet not only fights off these free radicals that cause signs of aging, but it also reduces inflammation of the gut and makes immune systems stronger than ever.

The healthiest way to stop feeding cancer cells is to increase healthy fats. Many who make the decision to limit carbohydrates in their diets make the mistake of increasing their protein intake. Too much protein will increase production of glucose via gluconeogenesis. I know I have written that many times, but it is such a common mistake that people make when cutting out carbohydrates. Limit protein to high quality organic and pastured sources only. In cancer patients, I recommend 0.5 grams of protein per pound of lean body weight, which averages around 50 grams of protein a day.

Myth #3: Low-Carb Diets Exclude Food Groups That Are Essential

If you want to become keto-adapted, you must remove certain food items from your diet. These are primarily starches, including grains, legumes, candy, sugary condiments, drinks, and other high-carb foods. Most people with damaged metabolisms must also eliminate fruit. Despite the publicity hype about all of these foods, there is no genuine need for them in the diet. Humans didn't have access to many of these foods throughout evolutionary history. We also didn't start eating grains until about 10,000 years ago, and we undoubtedly didn't start eating processed junk foods until very recently. Sugar used to be a very expensive commodity, costing ten times as much as milk.

There simply is no vitamin or mineral in carb-laden foods that we can't get in greater amounts from meat, herbs, and vegetables. There is no genuine need for foods like grains in the diet. In fact, grains are often considered to be anti-nutrients, which means they interfere with our bodies' ability to absorb nutrients. Grains, for example, are very high in something called phytic acid, a substance that hinders absorption of iron, zinc, and calcium from the diet,[21] Another benefit of avoiding wheat (including whole wheat) is that it can lead to improvements in vitamin D levels. This is because the consumption of wheat fiber has been shown to reduce blood levels of this very important vitamin,[22] Low-carb diets don't contain wheat and are low in phytic acid; therefore, they don't contain substances that "steal" nutrients from the body.

Have you ever noticed that kids get sick a lot from Halloween until Valentine's Day? Do you blame it on the cold weather? Guess again. There are holidays in between that time that focus on candy. Sugar depresses the immune system. Vitamin C is needed by white blood cells so that they can defend against viruses and bacteria. White blood cells require a concentration of vitamin C fifty times higher inside the cell than outside, so it is vital your children are getting enough vitamin C.

There is something called a "phagocytic index" which tells you how rapidly a particular lymphocyte can gobble up a virus, bacteria, or cancer cell. In 1970, a man named Linus Pauling discovered that white blood cells need a high dose of vitamin C. It was at this time that he came up with his theory that you need high doses of vitamin C to combat the common cold.

We know that glucose and vitamin C have similar chemical structures, so what happens when the sugar levels go up? Glucose and vitamin C compete for entrance into the cells. Additionally, the thing that mediates the entry of glucose into the cells is the same thing that mediates the entry of vitamin C into the cells. If there is more glucose around, there will be less vitamin C allowed into the cell. And it doesn't take much glucose, either: a blood sugar value of 120 reduces the phagocytic index by 75%. So when you eat sugar, your immune system slows down to a crawl.

Simple sugars also aggravate asthma; cause mood swings; magnify personality changes; increase mental illness; fuel nervous disorders; increase diabetes and heart disease; grow gallstones; accelerate hypertension; and magnify arthritis. Since sugar lacks minerals and vitamins, it draws upon the body's micro-nutrient stores in order to be metabolized into the system.

So, what are you sending your kids off to school with? A bowl of cereal and skim milk? A Pop-tart? To keep your kids healthy and focused at school, try feeding them organic eggs with lots of omega-3 and healthy protein, or my Shamrock Shake recipe. A healthy fat- and protein-filled breakfast is proven to increase focus and success in children as well as in adults.

Most natural, unprocessed foods that are high in fat like eggs, meat, fish, and nuts are incredibly nutritious and are especially rich in fat soluble vitamins, which low-fat diets lack. Not a single one of the studies on a well-formulated keto-adapted diet show any signs of a nutrient deficiency.

BENEFIT #4: Decrease in Undesired Side Effects of Menopause

If you're a female in your twenties, you may read this section and wonder why on earth you would ever want your period to come back. Well, our menstrual cycle produces hormones that create a snowball effect for many other desired processes that come along with it. Menopausal women often suffer from tissue dryness and decreased libido (not to mention their body temperatures are going through the roof and they often gain belly fat). During menopause, many of my clients complain they are losing some of their feminine features on their face and body and are taking on a more masculine appearance. This is because their bodies are mimicking masculine hormone production (less healthy estrogen and progesterone). And these undesired effects are just the external ones. Internally, there are some serious issues going on too, such as bone loss, decreased production of collagen and elastin, and decreased muscle mass. The unpredictable hormonal highs and lows, along with clothing not fitting the way it used to, can be shattering to a woman's mental and emotional well-being.

> **HEALTH TIP: Men can also have excess estrogen, which causes inflammation in the prostate gland.**

It has been grossly simplified that menopausal women have low estrogen; because of this simplification, these women are often given estrogen as a hormone replacement which can cause further estrogen dominance. The first hormonal shift for menopausal women is a downgrade in progesterone. Not estrogen. In some cases, estrogen levels get too high. Estrogen and progesterone need to be counter-balanced. When progesterone levels fall, estrogen levels shoot up to compensate, causing estrogen dominance. What causes low progesterone? Low-fat diets (specifically diets low in saturated fat) and external "bad" estrogens.

Our body produces three types of estrogen:

1. Estradiol (This healthy, or "good," estrogen is produced by the ovaries.)

2. Estrone (Fat cells store and form this unhealthy, or "bad," estrogen.)

3. Estriol (This type is produced only when a woman is pregnant.)

Healthy estrogen from our ovaries gives women ample curves, attractive breasts, and youthful skin. Unhealthy estrogen from our fat cells and external sources, however, causes too many curves (you might say "bulges") mainly in the belly area. Farmers have known this for years. They use a little synthetic estrogen to fatten their cattle. But women say to themselves; "I don't take any form of estrogen. Why do I have too much?" The sad truth is that estrogen comes from what we eat. Excess bad estrogen can come from several sources.

The following sections describe where excess bad estrogen originates from:

1. Carbohydrates and sugar. Our bodies make more estrogen when we eat too many processed carbohydrates. Insulin, the master hormone, is secreted from the pancreas in response to sugar and processed carbohydrates. Insulin stores fat and also causes our bodies to make more unhealthy estrogen.

2. Pesticides. Non-organic produce and coffee contain pesticides which are xenoestrogens. This would include herbs and spices.

3. Non-organic meat and poultry. Today, more than 80% of cattle are raised by using artificial hormones that help increase the growth rate as well as the body mass of cattle. These hormones are zeranol, estradiol, testosterone and progesterone, melengestrol acetate, and trenbolone acetate. Zeranol and estradiol can cause some serious health problems.

These hormones in food products can lead to severe health problems which include ovarian cysts and cancer.

4. Soy consumption. Soy contains "isoflavones" which are changed in the body to phytoestrogens (similar to the hormone estrogen).

5. Alcohol. Alcohol causes a quicker aromatization of androgens into estrogens, which explains why men who are heavy drinkers often get gynecomastia (enlarged breasts) over a period of time.

6. Plastics and microwaves. Make sure to never microwave in plastic or drink from plastic water bottles.

7. Topical products and soaps. Even common soap can be estrogenic, and anything you put on your skin will get absorbed into the bloodstream.

Despite some of the things you may have been told about the benefits of soy during menopause, I am not going to recommend it. Soy is damaging in too many ways and actually increases estrogen even further. Soybeans have a couple of issues. One problem is phytic acid, also called phytates. This is an organic acid (found in the hulls of all wheat) which block the body's ability to absorb minerals like calcium, magnesium, iron, and especially zinc. Soybeans also contain enzyme inhibitors called trypsin which block absorption of enzymes that the body needs for protein digestion and can cause serious gastric distress, reduced protein digestion, and can lead to chronic deficiencies in amino acid uptake (causing depression and other mood disorders and a decrease in muscle tone). Soybeans also contain a clot-promoting substance called hemagglutinin, which causes red blood cells to clump together. These blood cells are unable to absorb oxygen for distribution to a given cell's mitochondria (a process that allows us to burn fat when we exercise) and is detrimental for cardiac health. Trypsin and hemagglutinin are "growth depressants," a fact that explains why soy formula is so bad for babies. So, instead of soy, let's look into a different formula for menopause.

Let's discuss how having a low level of healthy estrogen affects menopausal symptoms. A well-formulated keto-adapted diet works for menopausal symptoms by replacing glucose that's lacking from the estrogen-deprived brain. When glucose can't get into brain, it causes hot flashes and low cognitive function, two common complaints of my clients going through menopause. Ketone bodies are water-soluble by-products of fat breakdown that can pinch-hit for glucose in the brain and other tissues.

When the brain is deprived of estrogen after decades of exposure, hot flashes arrive. During the years of exposure, estrogen becomes closely involved in the transportation of glucose into the brain cells. When we are menstruating and have healthy estrogen, this hormone transports about 40% more glucose into brain cells than what would be shuttled without estrogen. When the healthy estrogen goes away at menopause, the amount of glucose transported into the brain cells decreases, and the brain cells become a little starved for energy. The hypothalamus responds to this starvation by increasing the release of norepinephrine [adrenaline] in order to raise the heart rate, an act that increases the level of sugar in the blood; the combination of these events causes an increase in the body temperature. A hot flash, therefore, is an outward sign of the brain trying to protect itself from blood sugar starvation.

HEALTH TIP: Supplements can help speed up the estrogen-progesterone imbalance that women suffer from. Gamma-linolenic acid, or GLA, is an activated fatty acid that assists in keeping our hormones balanced. You can find GLA easily enough in food, but due to an overconsumption of trans fats, most people are missing the enzyme to convert GLA fats from foods. Instead, they must supplement with an activated GLA such as evening primrose oil which will keep skin soft and supple. We need those fats getting into the tissues. I prefer that women take 1,300 mg of evening primrose oil three times a day to help with hormone balance.

Ultimately, you want your body to use fat to fuel itself instead of carbs. Carbohydrates promote inflammation and lead to hormonal imbalances that further intensify symptoms. Menopausal women who halt the detrimental symptoms with a well-formulated keto-adapted diet often see a regular menstrual cycle return, have less belly fat tissue, and experience an increased libido.

BENEFIT#5:Fertility,Pregnancy,andaLow-Carb/High-FatDiet

So, I came to you just what, eight weeks ago? I asked for help with two matters: weight loss and infertility. I know from my measurements that weight loss is occurring, and we found out this week that I am expecting! How's that for fantastic news?! In just two monthly cycles, my body was able to do what it hasn't been able to do in three years (I started your eating plan on day 1 of the first cycle).

Many clients come to me with fertility issues and want help with getting pregnant. When women are eating a low-fat diet, this causes their hormones to not produce enough progesterone. Estrogen, progesterone, cortisol, DHEA, and testosterone are all made from cholesterol; if we don't eat enough, our bodies take cholesterol from our endocrine system to use for brain function and repair. When that happens, it's almost impossible for our bodies to maintain hormonal balance. When following a low-fat diet, what are women eating instead of fat? Carbs! Carbohydrates are metabolized into sugars which cause weight gain and insulin resistance, which in turn disturb normal ovulation because it converts healthy estrogen into androgens (testosterone). This is a classic sign of PCOS (Polycystic Ovary Syndrome) that I see quite often. Starch, sugar, and caffeine increase androgen production — it is because of this hormone that women often complain about dark hairs on their face and their inability to lose weight. Do not make the mistake of cutting carbs only to add more protein. Remember, too much protein turns into sugar via gluconeogenesis.

Saturated fats and cholesterol increase the production of healthy hormones, including thyroid hormones, which also help with fertility. We cannot have proper hormonal balance and conceive a child without adequate amounts of saturated fats. I often start my clients out with eating a "fat bomb" three times a day. A fat bomb is basically a tasty treat made with coconut oil, cocoa powder, and stevia. But if that is too rich for you, I also suggest stir-frying with coconut oil and using it in spreads like my "nut butters" (I always use it in my baked goods).

Cholesterol is so important during fertility and pregnancy: it is the foundation of normal cell function and it helps us digest fat-soluble vitamins like A, D, E, and K which are essential in the formation of healthy fetuses. Full fat dairy is also filled with healthy cholesterol, but I do find some clients to be dairy sensitive. For those particular clients, I suggest finding other sources of saturated fats such as coconut oil and quality animal fats, seafood, and egg yolks.

The following is a testimonial from a client who trying to get pregnant:

Maria Emmerich began helping me in my health journey before she even knew my name. About a year ago, I stumbled upon her blog [now named mariamindbodyhealth.com] and from that time on, I was hooked! Maria presents the truth about our health, our food, and the way our food impacts our health in a way that's easy to understand. Within a few weeks of reading almost every post on her blog, I ordered all of her books and began making small, healthy changes to my life.

Fast forward a year: When my husband and I decided that we wanted to become pregnant, I instantly thought of Maria as a way to help us naturally conceive. I had been experiencing some concerning symptoms and hormonal issues, seen various doctors and specialists, etc. and hadn't been able to find anything that worked. I wanted to work on balancing my body the natural way — with the food that I ate — rather than with prescription drugs, so I scheduled a consult with Maria and she helped guide me. We made changes to my nutrition and she suggested supplements that would help heal my body. Within a month, not only had my hormones balanced, but I found out that I was pregnant! It still feels hard to believe ... but I am so excited, so forever grateful to Maria for her guidance!

I will definitely be working with Maria and following her advice throughout my pregnancy and the birth of what I know will be a healthy, happy baby.

Thanks again for your help! I'm so excited! :) :) :)

—Kate

I get a ton of emails from clients a few months after these consults telling me how they are ecstatic and are now pregnant, but are wondering what to eat now. As if this diet of *real* food would be harmful to a fetus. There are many reasons why to not add in certain foods like gluten and dairy to a pregnant woman's diet. Many times, when cravings get the best of pregnant clients and they consume these foods, the autoimmune response results in a miscarriage. But even if clients are committed to staying away from gluten and dairy, they often worry that not consuming enough carbs is bad for the fetus. You will never find evidence of this, but you will read it all over the web. The information that clients read has a few flaws:

1. A huge mistake occurs when people (including doctors) compare benign dietary ketosis to diabetic ketoacidosis.

2. You can produce ketones in a starvation state. Instead of using a well-formulated low-carb diet, researchers starved pregnant rats to get them into ketosis. The flaw in that evidence should be obvious.

3. The last piece of so-called evidence is when they sliced up the brains of rat fetuses and saturated them in ketones. What happened was that the brain cells lived, but the brains stopped producing new brain cells. This is thought to be evidence that ketosis causes retardation.

Now let's dive into the facts. The lean human body is 74% fat and 26% protein (broken down by calories). Fats are a structural part of every human cell and are the preferred fuel source of the mitochondria, the energy-burning units of each cell. A fetus naturally uses ketones before and immediately after birth. Many studies done on pregnant pigs that are placed on ketogenic diets show fetuses with increased fetal brain weight, cell size, and protein content. In the early stages of pregnancy, there is an upsurge in body fat accumulation, which is connected to hyperphagia and increased lipogenesis. In the later stages of pregnancy, there is an accelerated breakdown of fat depots, which plays an important role in fetal development. The fetus uses fatty acids from the placenta as well as two other products, glycerol and ketone bodies. Even though glycerol goes through the placenta in small proportions, it is a superior substrate for "maternal gluconeogenesis." Heightened ketogenesis in fasting conditions, or with the addition of MCT oils, create an easy transference of ketones to the fetus. This transfer allows maternal ketone bodies to reach the fetus, where the ketones can be used as fuels for oxidative metabolism as well as lipogenic substrates.

During pregnancy, women become even more sensitive to carbohydrates due to an evolutionary adaption in which they become slightly insulin resistant; their bodies do this in order to allow a positive flow of nutrients to the developing fetus through the placenta. If the mom was more insulin sensitive than the fetus, there could be a nutrient shortage. Biology fixes this problem by making mom a little insulin resistant, effectively "pushing" nutrients to the fetus. This demonstrates just how important it is to feed you and your fetus a nutrient-dense ketogenic diet.

> **HEALTH TIP: I do not recommend losing weight while pregnant or breastfeeding. You store toxins in your fat cells. When eating a keto-adapted diet, you lose weight by burning body fat rather than lean mass, like you do with low-fat diets. For example, if you are losing one pound of body fat every four days, that is 3500 calories worth of toxins in your blood. Your bloodstream becomes very high in toxins since toxins are getting released from your fat cells. Passing them to your fetus or baby is definitely undesired.**

Breast milk is naturally very high in fat. If a newborn is breastfed, it spends a lot of time in ketosis and is therefore keto-adapted. Keto-adapted babies can efficiently turn ketone bodies into acetyl-coA and myelin. Ketosis helps babies develop and build their brains.

The following is a testimonial from a client who was having problems with a shortened cervix:

I actually went to the doctor's yesterday for a checkup, and you won't believe it. My cervix is back to normal! Thanks be to God! I'm still on

bed rest, but I wouldn't do anything differently now anyway. This [diet] is obviously working for me. Thanks again for your suggestions. I bought the prenatal vitamin you suggested and really like it so far.
—Dianne

I love it when my clients continue to consume those "fat bombs" they ate to get pregnant because the coconut oil helps with the baby. This is because coconut oil has antibacterial, antiviral, and antifungal properties which keep the mother and baby healthy. The extra coconut oil also helps with lactation, but more importantly, it increases lauric acid in the breast milk. Lauric acid is a rare medium-chain fatty acid found in human breast milk that supports healthy metabolism.

The following is a testimonial about a keto-adapted woman who had a successful pregnancy:

I just had a baby 8 weeks ago and followed Maria's woe the whole time. I occasionally went up to 60 g carbs a day because I love fruit and like to have it fresh and in season. I had the best, easiest pregnancy I ever had! I had very minimal morning sickness and less fatigue than with my previous pregnancies. I had no swelling and my blood pressure was perfect. I never experienced that extreme discomfort that so many women complain of. I 100% attribute a great pregnancy to Maria's way of eating. I gave birth naturally to a very healthy 7lb 5oz baby boy. I'm actually sad he's the last one because my pregnancy was so wonderful.
—Sue

BENEFIT #6: Elimination of Acid Reflux

In October of 2012, I started on the path to having gastric bypass surgery after years of yo-yo dieting and being overweight since around age 8 or 9. I did everything from doctor supervised [dieting] to phen-fen to WW to Medifast. My best weight loss was from Medifast, but it quickly became too expensive and it really was icky to drink shakes all day!

In January of 2013, I read a Wheat Belly *synopsis. This was an interesting concept to me so I bought the* Wheat Belly Cookbook *on Kindle. At the end of his book, Dr. Davis offered Maria's blog as a great place for recipes, guidance, etc. I checked it out and was impressed, so I bought [her]* Metabolism *book for my kindle. Then I had an initial health assessment and email consult with Maria. I immediately stopped my Diet Coke addiction (over 40 oz a day) — that was the hardest one for me. During this time, I started eating less wheat and sugar and by January 15th I got rid of all the grain products and went wheat free.*

Since that consult with Maria in early January, I've lost 51 lbs. The first 40 came off rather quickly, and the last 11 have been slower, but are still coming off at about 1 to 1.5 lbs a week. All this with little exercise (since I'm allergic to it! Ha!). I canceled my WLS that was scheduled for April 2013 and couldn't be happier. My moods have improved, I'm sleeping great, my body doesn't ache all the time, my hands and feet aren't always cold, I've not had a headache or acid reflux since late January, and my PMS is much better. I was experiencing facial ticks and vertigo type symptoms daily. The doctor didn't know why, but within ten days of getting off the Diet Coke, these ticks and symptoms were gone and haven't been back since.

I still have a long way to go (another 75 lbs maybe) but am now confident I have the right knowledge and the right nutritionist (Maria) to help guide me. Maria's books, blog posts, and Facebook page are great and full of eye-opening insights. I like most of her recipes I've made — especially the treats! I would love to be able to afford one-on-one consults, but my budget only allows for the basic health assessment and email consult. Of all the things I've done to shed the pounds, paying Maria (including books, cookbooks, and one seminar) was the best money I've ever spent. Wish I would have found Maria sooner — I would have saved a ton of money on wasted programs.

—Paula

Are you or someone you know taking antacids on a daily basis? Antacids cause ulcers, chronic inflammation, leaky gut, food allergies, anemia, inflammatory bowel digestive issues disease, and restless leg. Your stomach is a very acidic environment with a pH of 2 or less. Stomach acid is essential for absorbing vitamin B-12 and other minerals that allow you to release hormones from the pancreas, without which can lead to development of diabetes. It also helps breakdown protein. When you don't have stomach acid to breakdown food, undigested proteins sit like a rock in the intestines. This slowly eats holes in your intestines and the inflammation begins a detrimental snowball effect. When you start to have holes in your intestines, food starts to leak into your bloodstream (leading to leaky gut syndrome). This is awful because the immune system goes into overdrive to kill the unknown substances in the blood. This is what contributes to why we have food allergies! So if you have holes in your intestines and are a fan of cereal and skim milk, you will most likely develop a wheat, corn, and dairy allergy ... oh, boy! When this happens, other health issues follow, such as chronic/seasonal allergies, constipation and/or diarrhea, and inflammatory bowel disease (IBS).

It's important to understand that acid reflux is not a disease where too much acid is being produced, but rather it's a condition related more commonly to a hiatal hernia, a condition in which the acid is coming out of your stomach, where it's supposed to remain.

HEALTH TIP: A healthy thyroid produces stomach acid. If you are deficient in hydrochloric acid, you can't absorb the nutrients for bone health and thyroid function. Clients with thyroid disorders often complain of acid reflux, a "bump" in their throat, or trouble swallowing.

An organism called helicobacter pylori (initially called campylobacter), which causes chronic low-level inflammation of your stomach lining, is responsible for, or is at least a major factor in, producing many of the symptoms of acid reflux.

There are over 16,000 medical journals supporting the fact that suppressing stomach acid does not treat the problem of acid reflux. It only treats the symptoms. One of the explanations for this is that when you suppress the amount of acid in your stomach, you decrease your body's ability to kill the helicobacter bacteria. So it actually makes your condition worse and perpetuates the problem.

While you wean yourself off these drugs that suppress stomach acid (if you're already on one), you'll want to start implementing a lifestyle modification program that can eliminate this condition once and for all.

Here are some ways you can eradicate acid reflux:

1. Eliminate food triggers. People often mistakenly blame the spicy peppers for their acid reflux, but it isn't the peppers on the pizza … it is the crust and the cheese! The peppers are blamed because that they contain the flavor you taste when you have "verps" (vomit burps) — but that isn't the trigger causing the reflux. You need to start healing by completely eliminating items such as wheat, grains, dairy, and sugar. Excess carbohydrates also cause inflammation in the gut, which causes reflux to occur. It is important to also eliminate caffeine, alcohol, carbonated beverages, and all nicotine products. Soy and eggs can also be food triggers.

2. Eliminate all vegetable oils. Look at your packaged foods: most use canola, cottonseed, soybean oil, or corn oil. Even "healthy" mayonnaise, salad dressings, and roasted nuts contain these oils. Vegetable oils are very inflammatory.

3. Eat foods that heal the intestines, such as coconut oil, bone broth, and any "healthified" recipe that is dairy free.

4. Increase your body's natural production of stomach acid. Like I mentioned earlier, acid reflux is not caused by too much acid in your stomach — it's usually a problem with too little acid. One of the simplest strategies to encourage your body to make sufficient amounts of hydrochloric acid (stomach acid) is to consume enough of the raw material.

5. Eat sea salt. One of the simplest, most basic food items that many people neglect to eat is a high quality sea salt (unprocessed salt). I recommend eliminating the processed regular table salt for a lot of different reasons, all of which I've reviewed before. But an unprocessed salt like Celtic or Himalayan Salt will provide you with over eighty trace min-

erals that your body needs to perform optimally; these salts will also biochemically assist you to produce hydrochloric acid.

6. Take a hydrochloric acid supplement. Another option is to take a betaine hydrochloric supplement, which is available in health food stores without prescription. You'll want to take as many as you need to get the slightest burning sensation and then decrease this amount by one capsule. This will help your body to better digest your food, and will also help kill the helicobacter and normalize your symptoms.

7. Increase good gut bacteria. Eat fermented vegetables such as kimchi (recipe in chapter 10). You can also supplement with a high quality probiotic that includes bifido bacteria as well as acidophilus. This will help balance your bowel flora, which can help eliminate helicobacter naturally.

8. Optimize your vitamin D levels. I prefer clients to be in the 50-80 range of a blood test of vitamin D. Optimal vitamin D levels are essential for acid reflux as well because there's likely an infectious component causing the problem. Once your vitamin D levels are optimized, you're also going to enhance your production of antimicrobial peptides to 200. Doing so will help your body eradicate any infections that shouldn't be there. Tip: Always take vitamin K2 if you take vitamin D. Take 5000 IU with a meal (it is fat soluble) if your levels are tested below 50.

9. Implement an exercise routine. Exercise is yet another way to improve your body's immune system, which is imperative to fight off all kinds of infections.

10. Do not drink while eating. It dilutes your digestive enzymes that are responsible for breaking down your food.

Supplement plan to heal the intestines:

Ingest fifteen minutes to an hour *before meals*:

1. 3 grams of L-glutamine 30 minutes before eating. You can find this in a powder or capsule form. L-glutamine heals the intestinal lining and increases muscle strength. A healthy intestinal lining is essential for proper digestion, immune function, liver function, and overall health, primarily through its role as a barrier preventing the absorption of unwanted molecules. Glutamine plays a major role in DNA synthesis and serves as a primary transporter of nitrogen into the muscle tissues. It also decreases cravings of sugar, carbohydrate, and alcohol, helping you stick to the diet so that your acid reflux goes away.

2. Probiotics. A good probiotic should contain at least five billion live microorganisms per capsule. The ideal composition should include L. acidophilus, L. rhamnosus, S. thermophilus, and L. bulgaricus. These are considered "friendly bacteria." They are of great benefit to the health of the colon and to the immune system. Taken in conjunction with digestive enzymes, they balance the digestive system and reduce the possibility of acid reflux.

3. Digestive enzymes (one capsule before each meal). Enzymes are normally secreted by different glands in the digestive system, and help to break down food molecules into smaller particles in order to aid digestion. Enzyme production slows with age. Each enzyme has a specific function related to different elements of food. For example, lactase breaks down lactose (milk sugars), protease and pepsin break down proteins, and diastase digests vegetable starch. Those who suffer from acid reflux usually need more digestive enzymes than their bodies produce. A good digestive enzyme supplement should contain protease, amylase, lipase, cellulase, diastase, invertase, lactase, pectinase, and alpha galactosidase.

4. Aloe vera capsules. Add in aloe vera supplements. Aloe vera naturally and safely repairs damage done to the esophagus. Aloe vera buffers pH+ and it naturally speeds up the healing process.

Myth #4: Bad breath and ketosis

People who have been keto-adapted for longer than a few months do not have this issue, so why does it only happen in the beginning stages of a low-carb diet? I have a theory on this. When you go on a well-formulated low-carb diet, you lose a lot of weight, and it isn't muscle loss like many low-fat diets cause. You are losing fat. You store toxins in your fat cells. So as you lose fat, you are releasing toxins into your circulating bloodstream (this is why I don't like even obese clients losing too much fat while pregnant, since those toxins can be absorbed via the umbilical cord and passed to the fetus). The toxins, I believe, are creating a short-term issue of bad breath. After a certain amount of time, the toxins will no longer be an issue because your cells will be so clean and healthy. Stick with it — bad breath is a short-term problem of this awesome diet. You can also speed up the release of toxins by sweating in saunas or by doing hot yoga.

Bad breath is also linked to a vitamin C deficiency. Adopting a well-formulated diet after a lifestyle of sugar and starch can cause a vitamin C deficiency at first. If you have noticed an odor in your breath, I suggest adding in 500 mg of vitamin C a few times a day. You can only absorb a small amount of vitamin C at a time, so don't take 1500 mg all at once or you will just urinate most of it out. Eating parsley, which is high in vitamin C, can also help with bad breath. I hide it in my meatloaf, meatballs, and chili.

BENEFIT #7: Control Seizures, Autism, Epilepsy and Alzheimer's

I love all of the stories I hear about how clients lose weight and feel great on this diet, but when I get testimonies of children being healed, nothing feels better. Autism is a condition that I am seeing more and more in my office. Parents often come to me after their children don't have much response to other interventions and start to regress.

I put these children on a well-formulated keto-adapted diet, including a 100% gluten- and casein-free diet. I suggest medium-chain triglycerides rather than butter and cream as a primary source of fat. In one particular family, their son's childhood autism rating scale (CARS) score reduced from 46 to 15. If you are unfamiliar with the autism rating scale, I will tell you that this boy's numbers are so amazing: they signify a change from being severely autistic to being non-autistic. Not only did his CARS score improve, but his IQ increased by sixty points.

> **BAD BREATH TIP:** Grapefruit seed extract is refered to as "liquid gold" and helps immensly with anyone suffering from halitosis.

I really push a well formulated keto-adapted diet for my clients who suffer from epilepsy, seizures, and Alzheimer's (type 3 diabetes). This is because ketones aren't just fuel for our body, but they are also great for our brain. They help repair damaged neurons and membranes.

A well-formulated keto-adapted diet has numerous benefits for neurological conditions:

- It relieves neuronal starvation from cognitive hypoglycemia.

- It stimulates the essential immune response against intracellular pathogens, helping to heal brain infections.

- It eliminates an excess of glutamate. Feeding the ketone beta-hydroxybutyrate in place of glucose has been shown to cause less glutamate to form in the brain.[23]

  - This is significant because excessive brain glutamate is "excitotoxic" and kills neurons. Glutamate excitotoxicity causes destruction in a multitude of conditions including stroke, traumatic brain injury, spinal cord injury, and neurodegenerative diseases of the central nervous system (CNS) such as Alzheimer's disease, multiple sclerosis, amyotrophic lateral sclerosis (ALS), Parkinson's disease, alcoholism or alcohol withdrawal, and Huntington's disease.

- Epilepsy, schizophrenia, anxiety, and other mood disorders benefit from a keto-adapted diet because it decreases glutamate excitotoxicity.

Myth #5: I need fiber for constipation

Hi, Maria!

I have had troubles with constipation since I was six or even younger. I was in the ER constantly for pain and constipation all throughout my childhood and even adulthood. I would have to take ExLax often! I tried adding fiber [to my diet] and drinking water but nothing would work!

The pain is so severe from being constipated that I once thought I was consti-pated and ended up going to the ER only to find out I had kidney stones. From that appointment on they told me to use MiraLax. I used MiraLax for about twelve years, and when I read your [blog] post, I knew that I wanted to try the supplements and try and get off MiraLax. I tried not taking MiraLax for three days here and there and then would become constipated so I would always have to go back on it.

I have been taking the supplements you suggested for three weeks now and I am having bowel movements regularly. Just wanted to say thank you for your help!

—Amanda

Chronic constipation is uncomfortable and it is not healthy. Constipation is one of the most frequent gastrointestinal complaints in the US. There are at least 2.5 million doctor visits for constipation in the US each year, and hundreds of millions of dollars are spent for laxatives in just one year![24] If you are someone who thinks that it is OK to not go "number two" every day, think again. If you don't eliminate toxins and estrogens daily, they get re-absorbed and locked into cells, causing a toxic body and difficulty in losing weight.

Contrary to popular belief, fiber is actually causing more problems with constipation. I know you are reading this and thinking, "What!?" A diet that is low in fiber has been proven *not* to be the cause of constipation, and the success of a diet high in fiber is modest. There was a study done that proved only 20% of constipated patients benefitted from fiber. Further research points out that most patients actually suffer from worse symptoms when increasing their fiber intake. [24]

Beating constipation

1. Add in Probiotics. I prefer to start clients out on a bifido/acidophilus formula three times a day before meals (this will also cut sugar cravings). Once stool has normalized and the cravings are gone, I suggest a maintenance dose of one capsule a day. *Note*: Coffee will deplete the absorption of probiotics in the gut. Take them with water.

2. Add in Magnesium. Everyone has a different tolerance with magnesium. I suggest finding your magnesium tolerance with how lose your stools get. The type of magnesium will determine this effect too. Magnesium oxide is a very poor form of magnesium, do not buy this. I suggest a chelated magnesium such as Glycinate. I suggest 800mg about an hour before bed to help with calming you down and enhancing sleep. If you still are having hard stools with magnesium Glycinate, switch to magnesium citrate, which helps pull more water into the stools, thus helping with elimination.

3. Add in Vitamin C. If you are low in vitamin C, then constipation is bound to happen. I know that adding in supplements are so helpful in curing the problem. I suggest adding in 500mg vitamin C a few times a day. You can only absorb so a certain amount of vitamin C at a time so don't take 1500mg at once or you will just urinate most of it out.

The following is a testimonial about a client getting relief from constipation:

Hi, Maria! Thank you for your supplement recommendations! I added probiotics [to my diet] and it has helped me a lot! I'm actually down four pounds. I still need to add vitamin C and magnesium (I ordered them online, so I'm just waiting). But those probiotics work magic. I've taken antibiotics every year since I remember. I have always been ill with allergies, sinus infection, bronchitis, colds, etc. My friends would call me "Dolores" in high school; that's Spanish for pain. I was always sick and in pain. I've had constipation issues forever. I've taken fiber to help, but it never works. When I was desperate, Xlax was my way out.

Since [adding probiotics] last week, I've become regular. It's a miracle. My five year-old also has issues, and I started adding one probiotic pill to her milk in the morning. I open the pill and mix it in her milk. It's also helping her. Thank you, Maria. I keep learning so much by following you on [Facebook] and your blog and by reading your books, too.

—Angie

> **HEALTH TIP:** Are you or your children using Miralax for chronic constipation? This is not only not recommended for more than 7 days for adults, it isn't FDA approved for children! [1] Stop treating the symptoms and start treating the cause.

BENEFIT #8: Elimination of Candida (Yeast Overgrowth)

Maria, I wanted to tell you that I have had an unexpected benefit to eating your way. I haven't seen you address this before, and maybe it is a bit "gross," but for the first time in years, my tongue is pink! I can't remember the last time I didn't have a thick white coating on my tongue. I still have a long way to go, but I started eating the Maria Way about four weeks ago. I think I may have some additional allergies that I need to address, but I am working on it. Thank you so much for what you do!

—Argia

I just read a funny yet disturbing article on NPR called "Auto-Brewery Syndrome: Apparently, You Can Make Beer In Your Gut" (Doucleff 2013). The story is as follows: A sixty-one-year-old man was getting drunk in the middle of church. Strangely, though, he didn't drink a drop of alcohol that day! Sure, this Texas man did have a history of brewing his own beer, so was he still drunk from the previous evening? Nope, his gut was fermenting the carbohydrates he had eaten into alcohol!

One day, he went to the emergency room because his symptoms (including dizziness) were so bad. The nurses ran a breathalyzer test, and his blood alcohol concentration was a massive 0.37%. That is about five times the legal limit for driving in Texas. The medical staff basically blamed him for being a "closet drinker" at first, but a gastroenterologist and Cornell University wanted to really see what was going on.

They examined the man in an isolated hospital room for 24 hours; they gave him high-carbohydrate foods and would check his blood-alcohol (he started at 0%). At one point in this 24 hour period, it rose to 0.12%! Yep, he had his own Sam Adam's Brewery in his gut.

Essentially, this poor man basically had an extreme case of yeast over-growth, also known as candida. The strain this man had was called Sac-charomyces Cerevisiae. Eating a diet filled with starch, yeast, and sugar causes your gut to over-produce these organisms, which causes a bunch of issues (aside from getting drunk!).

Every body contains a sea of microorganisms, (bacteria, viruses, fungi) that reside in our intestines, throat, mouth, nose, you name it. Most of the time, these microorganisms do not cause illness, unless our resistance to them becomes lowered. Candida albicans is a yeast that lives in the intestines, mouth, throat, and genitourinary tract of most humans and is usually considered to be a normal part of the bowel flora. Candida enters infants shortly after birth. In a healthy baby, the growth of the yeast is kept under control by the baby's immune system. But if the immune system is compromised and weakened, problems such as thrush can occur. Candida coexists in our bodies with many types of bacteria in a specific balance. Healthy bacteria work to keep candida growth in check in our body ecology.

In a healthy body, the immune system keeps candida growth under control; but when immune response is weakened, candida growth can happen too fast. It is an "opportunistic organism" and will try to colonize all bodily tissues. The uncontrolled growth of candida is simply known as candida overgrowth. The first signs of candida overgrowth include nasal congestion, sore throat, abdominal pain, belching, bloating, heartburn, constipation, diarrhea, rectal burning or itching, vaginal itching and discharge, PMS, prostatitis, impotence, frequent urination, burning on urination, and bladder infections. If the immune system remains weak long enough, candida can also cause fatigue, lack of concentration, mood swings, dizziness, headaches, bad breath, coughing, wheezing, joint swelling, arthritis, failing vision, ear pain, deafness, tearing eyes, muscle aches, depression, irritability, sweet cravings, numbness and tingling, cold hands and feet, asthma, hay fever, allergies, hives and rashes, eczema, psoriasis, and chronic fungal infections.

The most common causes of candida overgrowth are antibiotics, steroids, over-the-counter anti-inflammatory drugs, oral contraceptives, mercury dental fillings, drugs or alcohol, chlorinated drinking water, meat or dairy products from animals fed antibiotics, and diets full of sugar and refined and processed foods.

If candida overgrowth is present, certain foods should be eliminated from the diet, and specific supplements such as probiotics (not more antibiotics) need to be incorporated. Even things like most vinegars must be eliminated. Coconut vinegar is the only vinegar I use in my recipes because it does not increase candida overgrowth.

BENEFIT #9: Elimination of Migraines

When clients come to me pleading for help eliminating migraines, I grin because to me it is an easy fix and I know they are going to feel wonderful soon. First off, you must drink half your body weight in ounces. Dehydration and not enough quality salt are main causes of headaches.

There are a few other major causes of severe headaches and migraines, and they all can be healed by a well-formulated keto-adapted diet. The following is a list of some of these causes:

1. Excess bad estrogen and low progesterone

2. Glutamate excitotoxicity. People with the common migraine tend to have a mutation in a regulatory sequence for genes that control glutamate abundance.[25] If glutamate excitotoxicity is the main cause of the migraines, then a well-formulated keto-adapted diet is a must!

3. Magnesium deficiency

4. Blood sugar issues

5. Food allergens

6. Low thyroid. Get checked by your doctor. You can also add kelp to your diet

7. Overcorrection with glasses or contacts. Get your eyes checked.

To help me determine what the trigger is for a client, I find out the frequency of the triggers. If these triggers are happening to a women during her cycle, then I know it is excess bad estrogen and low progesterone. Fat cells store and form unhealthy estrogen called estrone. In this case, not only do we need a keto-adapted diet to stop the excess estrogens from being produced, we need a diet high in saturated fat that is filled with coconut oil to produce healthy progesterone. Do not drink from plastic bottles, do not microwave food in plastic containers, and do not consume non-organic meats (they are injected with estrogen). I also find a huge connection between my clients with migraines and constipation. If you do not produce stool daily, excess bad estrogens get reabsorbed into the body; this process is the major cause of migraines in my female clients. We need to make sure to go "number two" every day or the bad estrogen will be redistributed instead of released from the fat cells.

The estrogen change during a woman's cycle can stimulate a migraine because the hormone change drops serotonin levels. Estrogen activates an enzyme called hepatic tryptophan 2,3-dioxygenase that shifts the metabolism of tryptophan from making serotonin (which makes us happy) to making kynurenic acid (which makes us not so happy). Women already have lower serum levels of tryptophan than men do (which may be part of the reason why we are more vulnerable to depression in the first place), so lowering available tryptophan in the diet with gluten and fructose may lead to even lower levels, which therefore causes depression.

In addition to the keto-adapted diet, I suggest supplementation of EstroFactors, evening primrose oil, milk thistle, magnesium, and if needed, 5-HTP to increase serotonin (only if not on antidepressant). This is a concoction for relief! See dosages at the end of this section.

If the migraines occur randomly or if you are male, the problem is obviously not an estrogen/progesterone imbalance (even though men can be estrogen dominant). In this case, the issue could be as simple as a magnesium deficiency. In such a case, a well-formulated keto-adapted diet will decrease issues with low magnesium.

For every molecule of sugar we ingest, our bodies use 54 molecules of magnesium to process it. And no matter where the carbohydrates come from, 4 grams of carbohydrates equal 1 teaspoon of sugar in our body. Let me say that again … 4 grams of carbohydrates equal 1 teaspoon of sugar in our body. With that thought in mind, let's look at some examples: A small Blizzard from Dairy Queen has 530 calories and 83 grams of carbohydrates, which equals 21 teaspoons of sugar. A 9 ounce bag of potato chips equals 32 teaspoons of sugar. Add a soda, that's another 16 teaspoons of sugar. With a diet this sugary, it is no wonder magnesium levels are depleted!

Magnesium in your cells relaxes muscles. If your magnesium level is too low, your muscles will constrict rather than relax, which will increase pain, including migraines or headaches. A magnesium deficiency can have serious consequences, including low serotonin. Since this mineral is necessary for the proper performance of serotonin, it is not surprising that many migraine sufferers have diminished amounts of magnesium in their brains. Serotonin is a necessary neurotransmitter that sends signals of satiety, satisfaction, and relaxation.

Insulin stores magnesium, but if your insulin receptors are blunted and your cells grow resistant to insulin, your body isn't able to store magnesium, so it passes out of your body through urination. To fix this problem, eat a well-formulated keto-adapted diet and consume high doses of magnesium glycinate.

Two other causes of migraines are blood sugar issues and food triggers. To combat the blood sugar issues, guess what I am going to recommend? Yep, a well-formulated keto-adapted diet. When your blood sugar is too high, it then falls too low, causing a migraine or headache.

I cannot emphasis these facts enough:

1. Carbs cause magnesium deficiency.
2. Carbs increase glutamate excitotoxicity.
3. Carbs increase free radical production.
4. Carbs increase bad estrogen, which decreases serotonin.

It is also important to focus on the health of our liver and kidneys to eliminate migraines. Again, drink half your body weight in ounces and eliminate all fructose to help get the liver as healthy as possible.

If you are adding magnesium, water, and quality salt to your diet and you do not have a thyroid issue, you could be having an issue with foods that contain tyramine. This is something I rarely see in my clients. But tyramine can cause blood vessels to dilate, and this may be what starts the migraine chain reaction in some people. Foods with tyramine can include foods that are considered good for a keto-adapted diet, so beware of the following:

- Anything aged, dried, fermented, salted, smoked, or pickled. Watch out especially for pepperoni, salami, liverwurst, and mincemeat
- Pickled, preserved, or marinated foods, such as olives and pickles, sauerkraut, and some snack foods

- Dairy and cultured dairy products, such as buttermilk and sour cream
- Aged cheese. If you get migraines, the best cheese for you is farmers cheese, cottage cheese and cream cheese.
- Vegetables like onions (may use some for flavor)
- Any fermented soy products (e.g., miso, soy sauce, teriyaki sauce).
- Nuts and seeds

The following foods wouldn't be on a keto-adapted diet anyway, but make sure to stay away from them:

- Fava or broad beans
- All alcoholic and fermented beverages
- Desserts or sweets
- MSG and related chemicals and products containing marmite, such as canned soup or bouillon cubes, meat tenderizers, seasoned salt

On rare occasions, nightshades will trigger migraines. This is important to note because nightshades are typically allowed on a keto-adapted diet. Nightshades include eggplant, tomatoes, sweet and hot peppers, eggplant, tomatillos, tamarios, pepinos, pimentos, paprika, and cayenne peppers (also potatoes … not that you would be eating those anyway, right?). Another trigger is tannins. Foods that contain tannins that are allowed on keto-adapted diets are avocados, vanilla, and cocoa powder. Foods that have tannins that you wouldn't eat on a keto-adapted diet anyway are aspartame, brewer's yeast, sourdough, dried fruit, red wine, caffeine, lentils, beans, papaya, passion fruit, pea pods, red plums, and carob.

In summary, if you follow a well-formulated keto-adapted diet, have plenty of water, and take supplements, you will be migraine free! As described in chapter 2, you may get headaches from a lack of quality salt in your diet. You need to get extra salt and potassium in order for your diet to be considered "well-formulated." I suggest eating homemade bone broth to get your extra salt and to get a hefty dose of minerals.

Supplements:

1. Three caps of EstroFactors with breakfast. This supports women with estrogen-related health issues by addressing multiple factors of estrogen activity and metabolism. It promotes healthy estrogen detoxification and elimination from the body, thus supporting overall hormone balance. Taking EstroFactors also helps to modulate pathways of estrogen metabolism, such as the conversion of estradiol to 2-hydroxyestrone, a weaker estrogen that may protect estrogen-sensitive tissues. It influences estrogen receptor function for more balanced estrogenic activity. Finally, it features L-5-methyl tetrahydrofolate a body-ready, nature-identical folate that is ideal for people whose folate status may be impacted by genetic variation.

2. Evening primrose oil (1300 mg at each meal, or 3 times a day). Evening primrose oil has been called the most sensational preventive discovery since vitamin C. It contains the pain relieving compound phenylalanine and is increasingly being used to treat chronic headaches. It is currently being studied all over the world as a treatment for aging problems, alcoholism, acne, heart disease, hyperactivity in children, symptoms of menopause, multiple sclerosis, weight control, obesity, PMS, and schizophrenia. Evening primrose oil contains a high concentration of a fatty acid called GLA, and it is this fatty acid that is largely responsible for the remarkable healing properties of the plant. The gamma-linoleic acid, linoleic acid, and other nutrients in this oil are essential for cell structure and for improving the elasticity of the skin. These fatty acids also help to regulate hormones (including the thyroid) and improve nerve function, aiding problems ranging from PMS to migraine headaches. The hormone balancing effect contributes to healthy breast tissue.

3. Magnesium glycinate (400–1000 mg per day). Do not buy magnesium oxide or citrate. Magnesium in its glycinate form is the most absorbable form and it relaxes muscles and tension. Many migraine sufferers

have diminished amounts of magnesium in their brains and since this mineral is necessary for the proper performance of serotonin this might show a connection between headaches and low magnesium. People with low magnesium levels find that their arteries constrict more.

4. CoQ10 (400 mg) increases the amount of mitochondria in cells, which increases circulation.

5. 5-HTP (200–300 mg). Take this at bedtime only, if you're not on an antidepressant. It increases serotonin. There is growing evidence that supports my long-term belief that migraines are a brain disorder. This idea, coupled with evidence of a "second brain" in the gut,might cause some to look at proper neuropeptide/neurotransmitter production by the digestive system as a root cause of the factors leading to migraines.

6. Two caps of silymarin. Silymarin 80 provides milk thistle extract standardized to 80% silymarin, which is noted for its antioxidant properties and support of healthy liver function. T4 is converted to the activated T3 in the liver, and the liver governs our moods and how well we lose weight.

BENEFIT #10: Elimination of Sinus Issues

A year ago, I met Maria Emmerich for a health assessment and consultation. My main goal was to lose a few pounds. However, I had also been suffering from IBS, allergies, and many sinus infections over the past several years.

Maria helped me change my diet and my life. She has a wealth of knowledge on how vitamins, chemicals and different foods can affect our metabolism, moods and energy levels. I would highly recommend her to anyone looking to make a lifestyle change, lose weight and get healthier for good, not just temporarily on the latest fad diet. The results will amaze you!

I have not had a sinus infection in twelve months and my IBS problems disappeared. No more allergy related eczema. And I lost weight (of course now have gained, being pregnant, but I'm smaller than I was with either of my previous pregnancies!). Feel free to ask me any questions. I highly encourage all of my friends to check out Maria's books and websites if you are serious about getting healthy!

—Connie

Congested sinuses, runny nose, and recurring ear infections are some of the many symptoms of a gluten allergy. Food allergies cause a variety of nasty symptoms because the offending nutrients are digested and absorbed into the body, and then dispersed throughout the body. Many people suffer from perpetual sinus problems, including congestion and blocked ears. I've seen too many clients be wrongly put on multiple rounds of antibiotics or even undergone multiple surgeries, but only experience subtle, short-term relief. Why didn't these treatments work? Because you are not looking at the cause, you are looking at the symptoms!

The following is a testimonial of a client with allergies and sinus infections.:

I started working with Maria about two months ago, but I have been on [a] low carb [diet] since January and I felt deprivation because I have a sweet tooth. Maria has saved me; I don't get my seasonal allergies like before. I would take Zyrtex, Flonase, Allegra, and I was still miserable. I would also get sinus infections and I had to visit the doctor for antibiotics. I notice I have not gotten my allergies. I may sneeze a little once in a while, but I'm not miserable like before. I know it has to do with my new way of eating, plus I've lost 27 pounds.

—Rachel

Gluten allergies are repeatedly overlooked as a cause of allergy symptoms. Let's dive into why eliminating gluten can clear up sinus issues without drugs or expensive surgeries. An allergy of any type is when the body's immune system responds to an "invasion" of a foreign product by generating large amounts of immunoglobulin E (IgE), an antibody that generates inflammation-causing histamine. Histamine causes inflammatory conditions such as sinusitis, which results in the production of mucous, leading to nasal congestion and sinus problems. Sinus inflammation can be caused by your body's response to gluten, if you have a gluten allergy. It can also be caused by a virus, bacteria, or fungal infection. This is why I always suggest everyone, including babies, take bifido bacteria. The health of your gut strengthens your ability to fight off viruses, bacteria, and fungus. If you already have a compromised gut due to celiac or antacid use, and a bacterial infection is the cause of your sinus issues, a round of antibiotics (followed by a hefty dose of good probiotics) will clear the sinus issues. If Candida overgrowth is present, sinus issues will most likely not clear up. Sticking to an anti-candida diet is also key to healing sinus issues.

If a virus is the cause, then the symptoms will resolve themselves over a short time. However, if your sinus problems are caused by an allergy, to gluten, for example, the only way to stop the response is to follow an on-going gluten-free diet.

BENEFIT #11: Asthma

I had allergy-induced asthma for nearly ten years and went to numerous doctors and pulmonology specialists. I would cough from post nasal drip for months of the year I was put on prednisone and multiple mess and inhalers. The very week I started your well-formulated, wheat-free, low-carb diet, my symptoms improved. After three weeks, no meds *were needed at all! This was a year ago, and I have never felt better!*
—Ann

The stem of all diseases is inflammation. What causes asthma? Inflammation of the lungs. What causes inflammation of the lungs? Sugar, starch, complex carbohydrates, gluten, and trans-fats.

Eating foods high in starch, even complex carbohydrates, cause the blood sugar to rise fast and then plummet to under the normal healthy level. The drop of blood sugar causes the production of serotonin to go down which causes depression. Then, the decrease of serotonin causes the production of histamine, which causes the expansion of blood vessels. Too much expansion of blood vessels causes liquid in the blood vessels to leak out. When liquid leaks out into the sinus area, it causes nasal drip. When it drips into the bronchi, it causes asthma. When it drips into the brain, it causes headaches and migraines.

The following is a testimonial about a child with asthma:

My family started eating [using] your plan. My youngest son, who is almost four, has battled the asthma cough and drip up until we changed our diet. Recently, we let him have regular pizza at a party. Since then, it's been cough, cough, cough, runny nose, and drip, drip, drip. Ugh! On day six I saw an improvement,, and on day seven, he finally lost the cough. It is amazing what eating the "Maria Way" can do, even for youngsters!
—Beth

I want to touch on asthma as it relates to food allergies, which can develop when food is not properly digested (this then causes fermentation activated by yeast in the intestines). One reason for the lack of digestion are the herbicides (like Round Up) that are ingested from genetically modified corn, soy, and other genetically modified foods. This process further increases the amount of yeast in the digestive tract. The increased level of yeast causes the increased penetrability of the wall of the intestine, which can cause "leaky gut syndrome." The undesired micro-organisms (yeast) enter the bloodstream and attack different parts of the body (lungs, vagina, kidneys, brain, and other organs). This can create asthma, yeast infections, allergies, sinus infections, chronic fatigue, and depression.

> **HELPFUL REMINDER:** It takes 54 mg of magnesium to process 1 gram of sugar or starch.

Many mineral deficiencies can also cause asthma. The mineral magnesium is possibly the single most important nutrient for managing asthma because of its multiple effects on the asthmatic condition. It plays an extremely powerful role in the relaxation of bronchial muscle, resulting in a reduction of bronchospasm and increase in the diameter of airways. Magnesium stimulates the production of AMP and ATP, two important mediators that create relaxation of bronchospasm. Magnesium also reduces the histamine response, which calms inflammation. Patients suffering from asthma often have high histamine release from white blood cells, which causes inflammation and bronchoconstriction. Magnesium will dull this response.

Also, a diet low in omega-6 fatty acids and high in omega-3 fatty acids will help. When that balance is out of whack, inflammation can set in. Eliminating all vegetable oils (which are high in omega-6) will help.

BENEFIT #12: Elimination of Chronic Pain

I wanted to offer a testimonial that has nothing to do with weight loss and everything to do with life! I have been in three bad car accidents in my life, so my whole back is bad, with very limited range of motion. My lower back and hips are fused and growing towards each other in a way they should never do. I am forty-four years-old and my doctors say I have the back "of an eighty-seven-year-old." This is my normal. I have taken 1–3 800 mg of ibuprofen for almost a decade. I also spend at least an hour of deep stretching to manage my pain. I only take what I must have and I have a very high tolerance to pain. While I have always hated taking ibuprofen, if I don't take it I literally can't get out of bed.

After taking the supplements you recommended, I have not taken any ibuprofen for six weeks! Just think of what that means to my whole system. Do I hurt? Yes. Can I get out of bed, work out two times a day, and have dance parties with my wee ones? YES! You have given my system, my life, and my babies so much and we are so thankful. All the knowledge you have and share, all the hard work you did and do each day specifically has given me a life I honestly never thought was possible.

—Lisa

When I was in high school, I volunteered at a nursing home. When I asked the residents what the secret to a happy life was, they often responded with "take care of your back!" At first, I thought it was a metaphor, but they explained that if you are living with pain, there is no way to focus on anything else in your life.

How many times do you take pain killers for a headache, joint pain, cramps, relief from strenuous exercise, or — dare I mention — a hangover (you all know how I hate alcohol)? Ibuprofen (also known as Advil) can cause some serious issues, especially if you have "leaky gut." If you tell your doctor that you have "leaky gut," they may dismiss your diagnosis. A lot of doctors claim there is no such thing as "leaky gut," but anyone dealing with IBS (Irritable Bowel Syndrome), Celiac disease, Crohn's, Colitus, or adrenal fatigue, know that is a true problem.

Even the New York Times writes about how ibuprofen causes "leaky gut." Every year, about 16,500 arthritis patients die from gastrointestinal damage due to non-steroidal anti-inflammatory drugs (NSAIDs). These pain killers are responsible for 103,000 hospitalizations per year. Vioxx and Celebrex are the newer prescription non-steroidal anti-inflammatory drugs, whose manufacturers claim they are better because they do not damage the gastrointestinal lining. As it turns out, they are wrong!

It has been proven that, over time, these medications also make your intestines become "Swiss cheese" (visualize many small holes in your intestinal lining). This permeation of the gut lining causes serious issues, such as allowing the protein in your foods (gluten in wheat, casein in dairy, and so on) to leak regularly into the bloodstream; this causes an autoimmune response because the blood doesn't like that stuff in there! It also allows small amounts of bacteria and digestive enzymes to get into the bloodstream. This is not a good outcome.

I get a lot of questions about the supplements I recommend, but people feel so comfortable about taking pills that are advertised on television. All of the supplements I recommend can be found in food, just in a "therapeutic dose." On the other hand, ibuprofen is not naturally derived but was synthesized by pharmaceutical chemists in the 1960s. The original synthetic route involved reacting isobutylbenzene with acetyl chloride to make 4-acetyl isobutyl benzene. This is converted in two steps to an aldehyde, which is reacted with hydroxylamine to an intermediate hydroxyl imine. This is dehydrated to the nitrile, which undergoes a final acid-catalyzed hydrolysis to ibuprofen. A competing pharmaceutical company simplified the number of steps later on using catalysts.

Instead of having my clients continue to pop pills filled with undesired properties, I prescribe them a variety of anti-inflammatory supplements that are natural and can be found in plant and animal sources (they are just condensed into therapeutic doses). Simply consuming certain foods with the pain relieving compounds will not provide enough benefit for someone in extreme pain.

Some of my recommendations include:

1. A high dose of quality fish oil. At least 1000 mg if not 2000 mg three times a day.

2. L-glutamine to help with muscle tightness. I recommend 2 to 3 grams three times a day.

3. Magnesium to help relax muscles that are extremely tight.

4. Two to three caps of Kaprex right away in the morning. Kaprex is a new and natural plant-derived supplement that effectively relieves pain and inflammation rapidly, without causing any adverse side effects. It features a specific blend of vitamin D, zinc, and selenium for additional immune support. There are other natural pain-relievers and anti-inflammatory supplements that are also safe, but according to board certified nutritionist Dr. Joseph Debé (on his website drdebe. com), Kaprex has been found to be 250% more effective than the best of those products. Both the non-steroidal anti-inflammatory drugs and Kaprex work by reducing the amount of prostaglandin E2 (PGE2) in our cells, but they do so through different mechanisms. PGE2 is a powerful hormone-like chemical that is responsible for producing pain and inflammation associated with arthritis and other pain-inducing issues.

I also put clients who have taken high doses of pain killers in the past on liver cleansing supplements. The liver controls our moods and cholesterol as well as how effectively we lose weight.

If you are an athlete that uses pain killers after strenuous exercise, pay attention. Pain killers inhibit your intestines from absorbing nutrients which help fill your muscle cells with the essential amino acids and vitamins which in turn helps with rebuilding muscle tissue. So please think twice about popping those little pills, and take fish oil to kill the inflammation instead.

Diet is key in healing inflammation and eliminating pain. A well-formulated keto-adapted diet alleviates pain and has an overall anti-inflammatory effect.[26] The initial indicator of almost every illness is inflammation of our cells. It is therefore critical for us to get a better understanding of what causes inflammation and to choose the right foods to prevent it from happening. Inflammation is usually associated with pain, swelling, and heat. But it doesn't always show externally: "silent inflammation" is dangerous because we usually don't know we have it until we fall ill. Everyday issues like headaches, sinus problems, allergies, skin disorders, acne, heart disease, stroke, aching joints and back, arthritis, and coughing are nothing more than a physical manifestation of silent inflammation. By the time we notice and address the symptoms, our cells have already been inflamed for a long time. One of the reasons so many people are dealing with inflammation is because of a rapid rise in blood sugar, which causes biochemical changes in cells. Choosing low carbohydrate foods is one of the best ways to decrease inflammation. When blood sugar rises, sugar attaches to collagen in a process called "glycosylation," and form damaging AGEs (advanced glycation end-products) which increase inflammation. A well-formulated keto-adapted diet (which is very high in healthy fats) give our cells the structure they need. This, along with a therapeutic dose of anti-inflammatory supplements, is the "secret to a happy life" according to my friends in the nursing home.

BENEFIT #13: Elimination of Acne

Acne is one of the easiest problems to treat naturally. Just like other chronic diseases running rampant in Western society (like diabetes, heart disease, and obesity), acne is primarily a disease of the Western world.

—Dr. Mercola (Chairman of the Department of Family Practice at St. Alexius Medical Center in Illinois)

Acne is much less of a problem in non-Westernized societies, where refined carbohydrates and sugar are consumed in much lower amounts. Solid evidence exists that diets high in sugar and refined carbohydrates are the primary cause of acne.

—Dr. Mercola

If you or your children are frustrated with acne, a grain-free diet will very likely clear up your skin. If you have been on a low-fat or "fad" diet, you may be also dealing with some vitamin or mineral deficiencies, so concentrated doses of supplements like vitamin A and zinc may be a necessity, too. Vitamins A, D, E and K deficiencies are common with low-fat diets; these vitamins are 'fat-soluble' meaning you can't absorb them without fat. A vitamin A deficiency is a major factor in acne.

Antibiotics are unnecessary and unsafe because correcting your diet creates an internal environment that does not allow bacterial overgrowth to occur. Taking antibiotics is very detrimental to your gut flora. It kills all of your good bacteria, a process that can lead to autoimmune diseases and food allergies.

> **FUN FACT:** You can decrease your child's chance of a food allergy by 70% if you give them bifido bacteria in the first year of their life. It is naturally found in breast milk if the mother is eating fermented veggies.

STEP 1: ELIMINATE "SIMPLE CARBOHYDRATES FROM YOUR DIET. We all know that "simple carbohydrates" are just empty junk calories. "Simple carbohydrates" include white bread, white rice, all sugars, soda, candy, and cookies. Eliminating these would be step one in clearing up your skin. Totally eliminating high fructose corn syrup is a mantra we all should follow. We need to teach our kids how to read labels and to never eat this. I found it in pickles! Fruit also contains a high amount of fructose, so it should be consumed in very limited amounts and never in the form of juice.

STEP 2: "COMPLEX CARBOHYDRATES" ARE JUST GLUCOSE MOLECULES LINKED TOGETHER IN LONG CHAINS WHICH OUR BODY BREAKS DOWN INTO GLUCOSE. Complex carbohydrates are found in foods such as beans, nuts, whole grains, and starchy vegetables. These sound healthy, right? But if acne is a problem for you, limiting these in your diet will decrease the inflammation of the skin caused by the rise in insulin. Our bodies prefer the complex carbs found in non-starchy vegetables instead of the complex carbs found in whole grains because our bodies each handle digestion differently. Vegetables, such as cauliflower, are slow to break down into simple sugars and have minimal impact on insulin levels, whereas the digestion of grain carbs, such as brown rice, raises your insulin. High insulin levels increase male hormones, which cause your pores to secrete more sebum, a greasy substance that traps acne-promoting bacteria. Insulin also causes skin cells to multiply, a process associated with acne. This rise in male hormones can also cause fertility issues, so a low-carb diet will greatly help women with PCOS.

STEP 3: IF STEP 1 AND 2 DON'T WORK, YOU MIGHT BE SENSITIVE TO GLUTEN. Gluten in wheat and other grains may be contributing to your acne symptoms if you have a gluten intolerance, which many people do. This is a separate issue from the insulin effects already discussed. Gluten is a prime suspect if you have rosacea. A person who is sensitive to gluten cannot digest gluten, so the body treats it as a foreign body when trying to digest it. The gluten can push the toxins through the skin and cause acne. But, you must be careful when choosing "gluten free" products; they are very high in carbs, which will not help your acne. It may seem impossible in our society to eat "gluten free" and "low carb," but we do it and we still enjoy pizza, donuts, and risotto (just in my "healthified" recipes in order to keep it ketogenic).

STEP 4: GET RID OF HORMONES IN YOUR FOOD. Get rid of milk, which has lactose and only buy organic hormone-free full-fat dairy products. Purchase hormone free meat, chicken, and eggs.

STEP 5: ADD IN HELPFUL SUPPLEMENTS SUCH AS COD LIVER OIL. Vitamin A and EPA/DHA are extremely helpful in clearing acne. Zinc, GLA, and other minerals can also help.

BENEFIT #14: Elimination of Eczema, Psoriasis, Rosasea, and Dandruff

After giving birth to my third child, I developed dandruff for some reason. It was quite frustrating as I've never had to deal with an issue like this. I did have dry skin but I've never had an issue with dandruff. I started using dandruff shampoos to help control it and none of them would work. In fact, it made my skin flare up with eczema. Ugh. You can imagine the hopelessness and frustration I was dealing with. It was horrible to be dealing with this brand new issue as a new worn out mom trying to take off baby weight.

Being such a good friend of Maria's, I felt comfortable enough to admit this to her, not knowing that she could even help with the dandruff issue. Immediately, she told me to try cutting out dairy from my diet. Wow, that is all? Well, I did it, and after two weeks, the dandruff was almost entirely cleared up. After those two weeks, it did come back, then slowly disappeared again. I eventually became dandruff free, eczema free and yes, I even lost the baby weight while following her low-carb, grain-free, high-fat diet.

Thank you, Maria! I'm so much happier and less stressed. It's amazing what a couple of bad food choices can do to our bodies and what good choices can help fix. I've never felt better than when I'm eating clean. You rock, girl!

—*Rebecca O.*

The most common strategy that doctors use to treat eczema are Hydrocortisone creams, which do reduce the inflammation a bit. The stronger steroids will reduce the inflammation even more, but not without side effects. However, the creams are not solving the underlying problem. All they do is reduce symptoms. They are just a "band-aid." Eczema is an autoimmune response. People with eczema appear to have inferior levels of a type of cytokine protein that's connected with a healthy immune system and have higher levels of a cytokine protein that's involved in allergic reactions.

I recommend eliminating common allergens such as gluten and dairy, as well as eliminating inflammatory vegetable oils. This often clears up the skin on its own, but adding in a supplement called GLA (gamma linoleic acid) clears the skin up even faster. Prostaglandins influence skin health and are the body's chemical messengers. They are created from the essential fatty acids that we eat, such as seafood. They are not stored in the body. This is why consuming essential fatty acids every day is so important. You can find GLA in foods, but due to overconsumption of trans fats, most people are missing the enzyme to convert GLA fats from foods and therefore must supplement with an activated GLA, such as evening primrose oil or borage oil, which will keep skin soft and supple. We need those fats to get into our tissue in order to heal the skin.

One of the easiest things I do for clients with eczema is suggest a probiotic supplements that includes bifido bacteria and lactobacillus acidophilus, which are healthy, good gut bacteria. It has been proven that children with eczema have low levels of good gut bacteria. By supplementing this lack with probiotics on a daily basis, gut health improves. When gut health improves, the immune system improves, and the inflammation on the skin is reduced.

I also recommend 1 tsp of cod liver oil, which contains vitamin A. A deficiency in vitamin A can cause dry skin and dry eyes. Taking 500 mg of vitamin E daily can also eliminate dry skin and itching.

Be aware that during the healing process, your body eliminates toxins from the cells that had built up, and eczema may reappear or get worse for a period of time. This process is normal and is known as a healing crisis.

SUMMARY:

The progress of modern biomedical research moves at a glacial pace; it needs decades to assemble sufficient evidence in order to get an application from skeptical reviewers to fund a clinical trial. People with brain (or neurological) conditions should simply experiment with a ketogenic diet themselves to see if it helps. Odds are good that it will. As I have shown in this chapter, the latest science is showing that a well-formulated keto-adapted diet can have a wide range of health benefits. Some countries are already recognizing this. Sweden recently adopted a high-fat, low-carbohydrate diet as their national policy for what constitutes a healthy diet. In America, it will likely take much longer to recognize this truth, but you don't have to wait. You can take control of your own health now and start leading a healthy lifestyle today.

Chapter 4

The Fat Switch

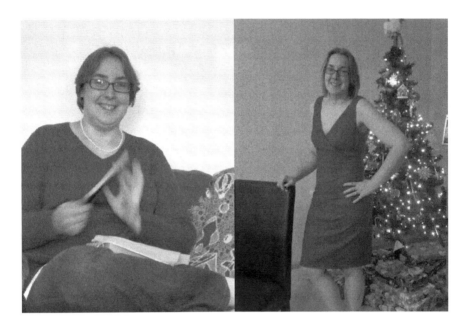

Dear Maria,

I had to write to tell you just how much you have changed my life. When I came to you for a consultation, I was at the heaviest I had ever been in my life. I was depressed, and scared for my health. Seeing my mom go through a stroke at age 57 ... I guess you can say it "scared me straight." I had been checking out your blog on and off for quite a while before I finally decided that I had to make a change, and I felt compelled to seek out your help. I was nervous, scared, and excited. I had tried so many different methods of weight loss over the years that I wasn't sure if this was going to work or not. Never in my wildest dreams did I think that my life would be transformed the way it has been because of all you have taught me. When I first met with you, we found numerous health concerns, besides being obese: I had a high estrogen level, sinus issues, severe eczema, asthma, intense cramps during my period, episodes of severe heartburn, and gas and bloating. Through all the changes you suggested and all of your amazing support, I am so thrilled to say all of these [issues] have disappeared. On top of that, I have lost sixty pounds, and I am still losing! I feel incredible, and I couldn't have done it and have kept doing it without you. Even after our month has been done, you have continued to be my number one supporter. Whenever people ask how I am doing it, I sing your praises. Many have asked to see before-and-after photos of me, and when I finally agreed, I was in shock. I knew I had lost the weight, but actually seeing it was unbelievable. I will never let myself get that size again. I not only feel great physically, but for the first time in my life, I am happy and confident in my body, and I'm healthy! You not only know what you are doing, you know what people need as far as care and support.

A million thank-yous,

—Leah

Fructose: The Key to Our "Fat Switch"

You wouldn't sit down and crack open a can of Mountain Dew for breakfast, but what if I told you that an 8 oz serving of Welches 100% grape juice (with the "No Sugar Added" claim on the front), has more sugar than a 12 oz can of soda? The worst part is that the sugar from the juice is in the form of fructose.

Fructose is a type of sugar that is the most damaging form of sugar to our brain and our cells. It causes metabolic syndrome and weight gain; this occurs not because of the calories, but because fructose turns on the "fat switch" in our bodies. Losing weight effectively and keeping it off requires turning off your "fat switch" and increasing the function of the mitochondria of your cells. As stated in an earlier chapter, the mitochondria are the "powerhouse" in your cells that are responsible for oxidizing fat.

The process of turning on the "fat switch" is as follows: When you consume fructose, it activates a key enzyme called fructokinase. In turn, fructokinase activates another enzyme that causes a cells to accumulate fat. When this enzyme is blocked, however, fat cannot be stored in the cells. Fructose is the nutritional ingredient responsible for flipping on this "fat switch," causing cells to accumulate fat.

Remarkably, this is the same process animals go through to fatten up in the fall and to burn fat during the winter. Metabolic syndrome is a normal condition that many animals go through to store fat to survive the long winters and migration. For example, in the summer, bears gorge on berries to fatten up for a long hibernation in the winter. In the book *The Fat Switch*, Dr. Johnson describes this process in more detail:

> For example, most animals have learned how to become fat and how to become thin. They do it in a tightly regulated way ... Hibernating mammals will double their weight and fat in the fall in preparation for winter ... I realized that I can learn by reading the studies about these animals. As I read them, I had another insight, which had not been appreciated before; these animals develop all the features of metabolic syndrome that we do. They get fat. They're visceral fat goes up. They get fatty liver. The triglycerides go up in their blood. They get insulin-resistant ... It's a normal process.
>
> It's not a disease. This is how animals store fat. It's part of the fat storage syndrome. I've actually proposed (and it's in press) that the metabolic syndrome really should be called the fat-storage condition, because it's just fat storage.[27]

Millions of years ago, our ancestors consumed fructose naturally from fruits rather than from the massive doses of high fructose corn syrup that we consume today, but they still experienced this fat-gaining phenomenon. During the summer, they would consume large amounts of fruit and would put on weight in order to survive the long, cold months when fruits and other foods were unavailable. This large consumption of fruit led to a genetic mutation that resulted in a greater uric acid response to fructose. Therefore, the more sugar we eat, the more uric acid our bodies produce, which increases our liver and intestines' ability to absorb sugar — this is a bad thing! Obese people absorb fructose effortlessly, whereas skinny people don't absorb it as well. [27] It is a detrimental snowball effect for my obese clients; the more sugar they eat, the more uric acid you make, which leads to further sensitivity to fructose absorption. Once you head down that path, it is almost impossible to stop. This is why I have to get so extreme with clients and tell them to cut fruit from their diets. If you start early enough and cut out all foods that are generating the fat snowball effect, you can recover. If you don't, you will lose the fat-burning, energy-producing mitochondria and you can't restore them. At this point, you reset your fat cells at higher metabolic set point, and your body wants to stay at that set point for homeostasis.

You can try and try to lose weight, but our fat cells have memories. They become cozy hanging out in your body and think they are protecting you. This causes the hormone leptin to misfire as well. Leptin and ghrelin are very important hormones that manage hunger and the feeling of full-ness. Ghrelin (produced in the stomach) increases appetite, while leptin (produced in fat cells) sends a message to our brain when we are full. An imbalance with these hormones causes us to intensely crave food and to never feel full. The worst part is that we never crave broccoli, we always crave high-calorie sweets and starchy foods. Over time, this imbalance can easily lead to long-term weight gain. Insulin, ghrelin, and leptin function as significant indicators to the central nervous system in the long-term regulation of energy balance, decreases of circulating insulin and leptin and increased ghrelin concentrations, studies prove that it leads to increased caloric intake and eventually contribute to increased fat cells during high consumption of fructose.[28]

In *The Fat Switch*, Dr. Johnson writes:

> The enzyme that makes you fat is turned on in obese people, and the enzyme that makes you lean is turned off. Once we realized that there was this switch, we asked, 'Why are people becoming obese?' Now we realized it was related to the sugar intake.[27]

The following is testimonial from a client who is bucking the status quo:

It's been two years and eight months since switching to a high-fat, low-carb [diet], and I've just passed the one-hundred-pounds-lost milestone! My lipids are the best they've ever been, with nice large, fluffy LDL [low-density lipopro-tein], low triglycerides, and rising HDL [high-density lipoprotein]. My IBS is gone. I can finally enjoy outings with the family rather than being tied to the bathroom! I have another hundred pounds to go to reach my ideal weight, but I'm feeling pretty confident that I'll get there in time.

I've been obese for thirty-four years. It is hard to believe it took over thirty years to find this kind of nutrition. Gary Taubes got me going with his books. It is folks like Maria that keep me excited and inspired nearly three years into this. Thank you for bucking the status quo!
—Jane

There is a very famous evolutionary biologist named Peter Andrews who works in London's Natural History Museum. He trained with Richard Leakey and is a world expert on human evolution. His research indicates that there are certain mutations in humans that occurred in our past. For example, we don't make vitamin C. We also have higher uric acids than most other animals. Andrews discovered that these mutations occurred during periods of human famine, and that they probably occurred to al-low us to become fatter in response to fructose than other animals. We're much more sensitive to sugar than most animals, and it's largely because of these mutations.

What is really scary is that a quarter of people who have fatty liver end up with scar tissue, and there is no recovery for them. These people can eat no fructose whatsoever. When they come to this point, they are suffering with cirrhosis of the liver. That is not because of alcohol, but it is from fructose. If one of the first three ingredients on a package of food is a form of sugar, you need to consider this food a dessert. Yes, even fruit. Sure, some people do not have a damaged metabolism and can tolerate some fruit, but I want you to understand that even in our days of eating Paleo diets, fruit was the sweet ending to a meal, not a "healthy side dish." If fruit had a label, the first ingredient would be sugar — this is what makes it tastes so sweet.

I can't tell you how many clients eat Lara Bars. Yes, they are gluten free and they are sweetened with dried fruit, but at 30 g carbs per bar, it turns into 7.5 teaspoons of sugar in your blood. That is way too much for anyone! And what about a "healthy" Chinese chicken salad for lunch? Since the first three ingredients are sugar, that salad should be considered a dessert.

We are programmed to love sugar.! That is because in our "Paleo days," sweet foods were safe foods: there was no poisonous food that was sweet. Many bitter foods were poisonous. Just think, how many times do you need to introduce an infant to a savory food? It has been shown that you need to give an infant a savory food about thirteen times before they like the flavor. [29] How many times do you need to introduce a sweet food to them? Once!

Fructose is an addiction. Many people would like to argue against this point. The brain, however, doesn't discriminate between substances: In the reward center of the brain, when you consume fructose or sugar, the dopamine receptors are stimulated. The overconsumption of fructose and sugar causes your dopamine receptors to downregulate, causing a larger "fix" to get the same high. It takes three weeks to break this addiction. And just as an alcoholic needs to cut all alcohol to break the addiction, you need to cut out all fructose in order to beat this detrimental addiction. You can't do it unless you know where it is hidden; that is the tricky part. An alcoholic easily knows what to cut out to beat his or her addiction and can avoid social circumstances where alcohol is present. But with a food addiction such as sugar, you can't avoid all social circumstances where sugar is present. You just need to be strong. Food and sugar is everywhere! Work, school, sporting events, family gatherings ... You need to be strong. I have more and more clients who are going to Overeaters Anonymous in order to beat their food addiction.

This addiction can not only give you a large waistline, but it also starts the snowball effect of memory loss and Alzheimer's. Sadly, I am watching my grandmother go through this right now. She is an amazingly strong woman who, after my grandpa died, decided to get her doctorate! She was always brilliant and loved to teach kids to read, so she went on to learn more so she could pass on her knowledge. She could have traveled the world, but taught kids instead. The sad part was that by the time she received her doctorate, her memory declined immensely. Alzheimer's is considered to be type 3 diabetes. It is metabolic syndrome of the brain. Insulin resistance is a precursor to Alzheimer's.[29] When Alzheimer's sets in, the brain can no longer use glucose for energy. It must use a different source. Enter ketones! Adding medium-chain triglycerides (MCT) in high doses multiple times a day, along with a keto-adapted diet, helps patients suffering from memory loss.[30]

Dr. Perlmutter, author of *Grain Brain,* has the following to say about Alzheimer's:

> This is a disease that is highly revenue-producing for mega factories of various so-called Alzheimer's drugs. The point is there is no meaningful treatment in 2013. It is a disease predicated on lifestyle choices primarily, because of the high amount of carbohydrates/sugar that we now, as Western-culture individuals, are consuming.

It's a preventable disease. It surprises me at my core that no one's talking about the fact that so many of these devastating neurological problems are, in fact, modifiable based upon lifestyle choices.

More and more studies are proving that large amounts of fructose in our body cause terrible damage to our bodies. The following is evidence of fructose's destructive nature:

1. A 2012 UCLA study showed that a diet containing steadily high levels of fructose actually slowed brain function, hampering memory, and learning.[31]

2. A 2010 Princeton University study demonstrated that fructose causes significant weight gain, increases levels of abdominal fat, and produces a high level of triglycerides.[32, 44]

3. A 2012 Duke University study showed that high-fructose diets increases the risk of ATP depletion. ATP (adenosine triphosphate) is a co-enzyme necessary for cellular metabolism, and when depleted, it triggers liver damage including scarring, inflammation, and non-alcoholic fatty liver disease.[33]

4. The American Journal of Clinical Nutrition reports that, along with ATP deletion, high fructose consumption can cause metabolic syndrome (because it generates uric acid), can cause dysfunction of the endothelium (the inner lining of blood vessels), can lead to the formation of fats (lipogenesis), and can cause oxidative stress and damage. They further report that fructose consumption may interfere with hormones that communicate satiety.[34]

Why Fructose Is so Harmful:

1. Fructose can only be metabolized by the liver. Glucose, on the other hand, can be metabolized by every cell in the body. Fructose raises triglycerides (blood fats) like no other food. Fructose bypasses the enzyme phosphofructokinase, which is the rate-limiting enzyme for glucose metabolism. Fructose is shunted past the sugar-regulating pathways and into the fat-formation pathway. The liver converts this fructose to fat, which, unfortunately, remains in the liver; this is the cause of fatty liver disease. Consuming fructose is essentially consuming fat. This is why I see so many children with fatty liver disease ... they aren't drinking alcohol, they are drinking sodas and juices and are consuming too much fructose!

In his book *Cholesterol Clarity*, Jimmy Moore says the following on how to remember that eating carbohydrates is essentially equal to eating fat: "One way to remember that eating carbohydrates leads to an increase in blood and liver fat is to compare it to the French delicacy foie gras, a "fatty liver," created by force-feeding carbohydrate (corn, or in Roman times, figs, which both turn into high amounts of fructose) to a goose. The same thing happens in humans."[59]

2. Fructose reduces the sensitivity of insulin receptors, which causes type 2 diabetes. Insulin receptors are the way glucose enters a cell to be metabolized. Our cells become resistant to the effects of insulin and as a result, the body needs to make more insulin to handle the same amount of glucose. We also start to produce insulin as a defense mechanism even if we don't eat sugar or starch. Yikes! This is why we shouldn't allow our children to eat so much sugar and starch either. Even though they may be thin and active now, you are setting them up for a future where they can't enjoy a dessert without feeling the negative effects. I grew up on Fruity Pebbles and skim milk for breakfast, and Cocoa Pebbles for dinner, which is why I am so sensitive to glucose.

3. Fructose is high in uric acid, which increases blood pressure and causes gout.

4. Fructose increases lactic acid in the blood. High levels of this acid cause metabolic acidosis, especially for those with conditions such as diabetes.

5. Fructose accelerates oxidative damage and increases aging. It changes the collagen of our skin, making it prone to wrinkles.

6. High consumption of fructose leads to mineral loss, which can lead to low bone density (osteroporosis). Such minerals include iron, calcium magnesium, and zinc. Fructose also interferes with copper metabolism. This interference prevents collagen and elastin—connective tissues that hold the body together—from forming. A deficiency in copper can also lead to infertility, bone loss, anemia, defects of the arteries, infertility, high cholesterol levels, heart attacks, and an inability to control blood sugar.

7. Fructose has no effect on our hunger hormone ghrelin, but interferes with our brain's communication with leptin, which is the hormone that tells us to stop eating. Unfortunately, you *can* become leptin resistant.

Fructose and Glycation

One of the big contributors to the aging process and the development and perpetuation of degenerative diseases is Advanced Glycation End-products (AGEs). Glycation is when a chemical reaction occurs between proteins and either sugars, lipid peroxidation products (free radicals from oxidative damage), or the breakdown products of sugar. So sugar plays a big role in glycation as does oxidative damage (think PUFA oils and sugar inflammation).

Glycation is the forming of sort of a crust around our cells. Many different studies have shown that this crust contributes to a wide range of diseases including diabetes, Alzheimer's, heart disease, asthma, stroke, cataracts, glaucoma, PCOS, autoimmune disease, and much more.

So what role does fructose play here? Studies have shown that fructose enables glycation reactions ten times more rapidly than glucose![35]

FINDING FRUCTOSE

Fat is the fuel, but sugar, and in particular, fructose, is the fire. Foods rich in fructose can activate the fat switch — resulting in loss of appetite control and a reduction in energy.

—Richard J. Johnson, author of *The Fat Switch*

Sources of fructose:

- Table sugar = 50% fructose
- Honey = 55% fructose
- High-fructose corn syrup = 55–65% fructose (depending on the brand)
- Agave = Can be up to 92% fructose!
- Fruits = Depends on the fruit, but apples are 70% fructose!

Where do we find fructose? We can find it in many foods, including the following: fruit, high-fructose corn syrup (isoglucose), high-fructose glucose, any concentrated fruit juice, any fruit syrup, beet sugar, corn sugar, brown rice syrup, brown sugar, date sugar, grape syrup, maple syrup, molasses, polydextrose, sorbitol, turbinado, inverted sugar (reducing sugar), inverted sugar syrup (also known as trimoline), sucrose syrup, golden syrup, honey, agave syrup, carob powder, Gur or Jaggery, panela, and rapadura.

Honey

It's no secret that white sugar is a food you should consume sparingly, but is honey a healthier alternate? Honey may be less refined and more natural than white sugar, but honey is still high in calories and fructose. It contains sugar and calories just like any other sweetener. One teaspoon of natural honey contains 22 calories. Honey actually contains more calories than sugar, as one teaspoon of sugar contains 16 calories. The biggest problem with honey is that it is roughly 50% fructose.

Although honey is a fattening food, it does provide some nutritional benefits that are lacking in white sugar. Honey contains vitamins such as niacin, riboflavin, thiamine and vitamin B6, though it contains only traces of these minerals. Additionally, honey doesn't even get close to the U.S. Department of Agriculture's recommended daily standards. Although these trace vitamins might make honey a slightly better choice than white sugar, it's still not a healthy food. Despite the fact that several websites claim honey to be some kind of miracle food, most of these statements are mythical and unproven. If you still think honey is worth using in your baked goods because of the vitamins, let me put it another way: only 2% of honey contains vitamins! And in most cases, store bought honey doesn't even contain the pollen that is claimed to have health benefits.[36]

Honey without pollen is a watered down, synthetic scam. The majority of honey on supermarket shelves is made from an ultra-filtering process that heats honey to high temperatures, using high levels of pressure to force it through exceptionally small filters to eliminate pollen. Why are they doing this? It is so manufacturers can hide where they are getting the honey from. And why would they want to conceal the honey's source? Well, because most of the honey comes from Chinese markets that are responsible for allowing dangerous antibiotics and ample amounts of heavy metals to enter imported honey products.[37]

You might be thinking, "OK Maria, then I will only buy honey from my friends who make their own." In that case, remember that by weight, a homemade batch of honey is 82% sugar. Half of that sugar (40% of the total weight) is fructose, and the honey still contains only trace amounts of vitamins and minerals.[38] Your body doesn't care whether you ingest honey or table sugar; once they enter your bloodstream, you produce an abundance of insulin. To your body, sugar is sugar. All types of sugar should be consumed cautiously, even if it is honey.

Coconut Sugar

Coconut sugar is a sweetener that has become very popular in the past few years. Man, I get a million questions about this sweetener. This sugar is derived from the coconut palm tree and is hyped as being more nutritious and lower on the glycemic index than sugar. Coconut sugar is made in a two-step process:

1. A cut is made on the flower of the coconut palm, and the liquid sap is collected into containers.

2. The sap is placed under heat until most of the water in it has evaporated.

Coconut sugar does maintain some of the nutrients found in the coconut palm. It is difficult to find exact data on this, but according to the Philippine Department of Agriculture, coconut sugar contains several nutrients. [39] Most notable of these are the minerals iron, zinc, calcium, and potassium, along with some polyphenols and antioxidants that may also provide some health benefits. The reason it is lower on the glycemic index is because it also contains a fiber called inulin, which may slow glucose absorption.[40]

Even though coconut sugar does contain some nutrients, you'd have to eat a ridiculous amount of it to really get any benefits from these nutrients. You would get a lot more from non-sweet foods. Coconut sugar has the same amount of empty calories as table sugar. So again, you may be thinking, "OK Maria, if I want to sweeten something a little, I will use coconut sugar since it seems less harmless than honey." No! Let me surprise you with a tidbit: even though I see claims all over the web that coconut sugar is commendably fructose-free, 70 to 80% of it is made of sucrose, which is half fructose (and half glucose)![41] This essentially means that coconut sugar supplies the same amount of fructose as regular sugar, gram for gram. As long as you understand just how detrimental fructose is not only to your waist line, but also to the overall health of your cells and liver, you see that coconut sugar should be avoided.

Agave

Agave's reputation for being a health food has finally fallen a little. I use to be laughed at years ago when I would tell people agave is not healthy and is terrible for your liver. People didn't want to listen to me because they would see it glorified on the Food Network's shows and commercials. It is so expensive, too, that it must be healthier than sugar, right? Even the name "agave" conjures up images of idealistic tropical expeditions and magical medicine.

A few years back I received an amazingly large and heavy box. It must have cost a fortune to ship. It was a box from a popular agave manufacturer that contained all of their products. My mouth dropped open. There must have been thirty bottles of various agave syrups. Strawberry flavored, cinnamon flavored, blue agave, dark, light … you name it, it was in there! What was I to do with this junk? I couldn't give it to a food shelf, I would feel too guilty. I had an idea to put it in my hummingbird feeders, but that also wasn't recommended when I researched it. In the trash it went.

If you're diabetic, you've likely been especially targeted and told that agave is the best thing that has happened to you since locally grown organic kale. You've likely been told that agave has a "low glycemic index," which doesn't spike your blood sugar. While agave syrup *is* low on the glycemic index, so is Crisco; that doesn't mean it's good for you. The reason agave is publicized as being "low glycemic" is due to the shockingly high concentration of fructose. It is 90% fructose and 10% glucose, a percentage that is far higher than even the demonized high-fructose corn syrup. As well, agave contains about 60 calories per tablespoon, compared to 40 calories for a tablespoon of table sugar.

Although the industry wants you to believe that agave nectar comes straight from the plant and into your jar, nothing could not be further from the truth. Despite manufacturers' statements, most agave "nectar" is not made from the sap of the agave plant but from its root.[42] The root has a complex carbohydrate called inulin, which is made up of fructose molecules. The process that most agave manufacturers use to convert this inulin into "nectar" is just like how cornstarch is transformed into high-fructose corn syrup.[42]

Agave is transformed into fructose-filled liquid through the use of chemicals and genetically altered through the use of caustic acids, clarifiers, and filtration chemicals.[42] Some of these chemicals include activated charcoal, cationic and ionic resins, Clarimex, Dicalite, hydrofluoric acid, and Fructozyme. The result is a highly refined fructose syrup, along with some remaining inulin. Yikes! Now do you understand why I couldn't donate that box of agave?

Fruit

Sure, I eat fruit. I eat a ton of avocado, tomatoes, lemons, and limes. But that's it, I never eat fruit. Fruit tastes sweet for a reason. I can already hear the critics as I write this. Yes, I am extreme, but that is why I have the results with clients. The fact that some very popular diets consider fruit a "free food" is ridiculous! When fellow nutritionists and health magazines suggest eating sugar to "cut your sugar cravings," I find it preposterous!

So if fructose is bad and fructose is found mainly in fruits, does that mean we should avoid fruits? Let's look at the percentage of fructose in some common fruits, compared to equal portions of honey and other products.

Item	Grams of fructose per 100 grams
Agave	65–90
High Fructose Corn Syrup	55
Honey	40–50
Dates	32
Raisins	30
Figs	23
Berry Jams (apple, blueberry, strawberry, etc.)	15–30
Dried fruit (peaches, plums, apricots, etc.)	13.5
Molasses	13
French dressing (reduced fat)	13
Catsup (or Ketchup)	9.3
Blueberries, wild	9
Grapes (red or green)	8
Pineapple	7.2
Pears	6.2
Apples	5.9
Bananas	4.9

Fructose becomes a metabolic poison when you consume more than 25 grams a day. You may be looking at the chart and mistakenly think that I am allowing you to eat any fruit, as long as you are under 25 grams, right? Wrong. If you are already having issues with metabolic syndrome, 25 grams is going to be way too much.

Check out the amounts on the apples and dried fruits. They have high amounts of fructose. Does that mean they're the devil? Not necessarily. But I do want you to be aware that fruit is sweet because it contains a lot of sugar, including a lot of fructose, which is so damaging to our bodies. Do not mistakenly eat fruit in abundance, believing it is a "free food." I just finished reading a book called, *Heavy*, which was a memoir of a mother trying to help her eight-year-old lose weight. In the story, the mother went to a dietitian who assigned colors to foods to help her daughter understand what foods she could eat without guilt, what foods she must eat in moderation, and what foods that she should not eat. Fruit was a food she could eat without guilt. So when the daughter wasn't losing weight, the mother desperately only fed her daughter fruit for breakfast. Since her daughter was always hungry on this fat-devoid diet, she would give her fruit for snacks, too. No wonder the poor little eight-year-old was always hungry! I loved this book and hated it at the same time. I loved it because it discussed what I see daily in clients and it reminded me of how I mistakenly followed that type of diet. I hated it because I wanted so desperately to call this mother and help her to stop creating an eating disorder for such a young child.

Another reason to limit fruit intake is that it is not the same as what our ancestors ate. Have you seen or tasted strawberries in the wild? My family has a strawberry patch, and the strawberries are about the size of the tip of your thumb and are quite tart. If you buy strawberries at Sam's Club, for example, they are larger than a golf ball and taste like candy, but that isn't sweet enough for most people. My niece once poured my dad's homemade maple syrup all over her bowl of Sam's Club strawberries, an act she was applauded for; eating fruit instead of junk food. I just bit my tongue.

We are breeding nutrition out of "natural" foods. I guess grapes aren't sweet enough for us anymore because we now have "cotton candy" grapes! These grapes are bred to have twice as much sugar as regular sugar-filled grapes.[43]

A lot of Americans are ingrained with the idea that they should be eating an apple a day, so they pick a big red Golden Delicious and feel like they are doing their "body good." But, hey, don't you know that Golden Delicious apples are a hundred-year heirloom? Shouldn't heirlooms be better for us since we can breed more phytonutrients into it? Not necessarily. Many times we focus on taste, or should I say sugar content, to stimulate sales. In her book *Eating on the Wild Side*, Jo Robinson reviews a 2009 study that examined forty-six overweight men with high cholesterol and triglycerides who agreed to participate in an eating experiment. Half of the men stayed on their regular diets, serving as a control group. The other twenty-three added a Golden Delicious apple to their fare. The goal was to determine if eating an apple a day would reduce the risk of cardiovascular disease. At the end of the study, the men who ate an apple a day had higher levels of triglycerides and LDL cholesterol than before the study began. The conclusion is that the Golden Delicious apples were too low in phytonutrients to lower the men's bad cholesterol, and were too high in sugar, causing an increase in the men's triglycerides.[28]

Fructose Intolerance and Malabsorption

More and more clients are coming into my office with even more difficulty with fructose than the problems listed above. Some people are born without the necessary enzyme, called aldolase B, to break down fructose. This congenital ailment is known as hereditary fructose intolerance or fructose malabsorption. This condition causes a build-up of dangerous substances in the liver and throughout the body if a person consumes fructose. The absorption of fructose is impaired by deficient fructose carriers in the small intestine's enterocytes. This means that the ability to digest fructose is impaired, and fructose travels down to the colon undigested.

When anything travels down the large intestine without being broken down, it causes some seriously uncomfortable issues. It immediately causes gas, bloating, pain, and diarrhea. But it also causes anger, low moods, rashes, acne, and colic in babies. Some of these symptoms can be quite embarrassing if they happen at the wrong time. I had a marathoner client who had a very embarrassing experience while running the Twin Cities Marathon after consuming a banana at mile eighteen. I will let you use your imagination.

> **HEALTH TIP: A damaged liver causes low moods and can lead to serious depression. Are you depressed? Get your liver checked and eliminate all foods that bog down your liver.**

Clients with fructose intolerance need to avoid all fructose, including all fruit, some vegetables, honey, table sugar, agave nectar, juices, sports drinks, and sodas. Consuming foods containing fructose can cause serious damage to the liver and kidneys if you don't eliminate sugar from your diet.

Fructose and the Paleo Diet

With a malabsorption issue, even the Paleo diet can be a problem. A lot of clients come to me and say they don't know why they don't feel amazing like the rest of their family does on the Paleo diet that they have adopted. Paleo is great for many reasons: it eliminates grains and dairy, but for 30-50% of Europeans and 15-20% of Americans, the low-starch Paleo approach encourages eating more fruit and things like sweet potatoes, foods that intensify many digestive, mood, and skin problems.

The Best Sweetener Choices

1. STEVIA. I prefer stevia glycerite over all other types of stevia because it has a non-bitter aftertaste. It has a thick, honey-like consistency. People tend to overuse powders, where the sweetness is really concentrated, so if you've tried powders in the past and didn't like them, try liquid forms. Stevia contains zero calories, but one downfall is that it doesn't work well for baking.

Watch out for hidden sugars in stevia brands like Stevia in the Raw, which contains maltodexterin. True, maltodexterin isn't technically sugar, but it is derived from corn. Sugar has a glycemic index of 52, whereas maltodexterin has a glycemic index of 110!

2. SOME SUGAR ALCOHOLS. Popular sugar alcohol sweeteners include xylitol and erythritol, which are natural sweeteners made through a fermentation process of vegetables or sugar cane. They contain fewer calories than sweeteners like pure sugar and honey, but more calories than stevia. They also leave a cooling sensation in the mouth and have been found to prevent cavities. In some of my clients who have damaged intestinal lining, too much sugar alcohol can cause GI distress. And it is very important to note that xylitol is extremely toxic to dogs. Even a little bit causes life-threatening changes in a pooch's blood sugar (as do grapes, raisins, onions, and chocolate).

If you or your kids are new to stevia and natural, low-fructose sweeteners, I suggest trying xylitol. It has the most similar taste to sugar. At least *I* think it does — then again, I haven't had sugar in a decade!

3. YACON SYRUP. Yacon is less than 1 on the glycemic index. It is mostly made up of non-digestible fructooligosaccharides (similar to the chicory root extract used in Swerve). It is a great option when you need a brown sugar or molasses flavor. It does have a small amount of fructose, so using it in moderation is important (typically I use 1 teaspoon in a 2 quart batch of ketchup).

NO Fruit? How Will I Get Nutrients?

We need to update the recommendation of eating nine servings of fruits and vegetables for maximum health. This suggestion has a few issues with it. A few years ago, I read that most kids actually do get the recommended servings for fruits and vegetables. Are you shocked to read this? Yep, they eat French fries, onion rings, and ketchup. Sad, but it does fit the guidelines. Will you reap the benefits of eating 7–9 servings of these foods? Absolutely not.

Even if you aren't even eating French fries or ketchup, eating three bananas a day isn't a good idea. Studies prove that the current state of the produce we consume is relatively low in phytonutrients, and much higher in sugar than it was in our Paleo days.[44] All of the fruits and vegetables displayed in our supermarkets have much fewer nutrients than what you would find in the wild. Consumers want fruit that tastes sweet. The sad part is, we think it is a good thing when our kids eat massive amounts of fruits. The more palatable our produce has become, the less beneficial it is for our health. The most beneficial phytonutrients have a bitter, sour, or astringent taste.

When I am asked if I eat fruits, I jokingly say of course! As I mentioned earlier, I eat avocado, olives, and tomatoes! But most people think I am a bit extreme when I limit most vegetable consumption for my clients, too. To get keto-adapted, even low-starch vegetables may keep someone with a damaged metabolism out of ketosis. So I limit vegetables to only red leaf lettuce, cabbage, cucumber, celery, and zucchini. I am also a huge fan of organic leafy green plants, herbs, and spices.

> **HEALTH TIP:** Organic herbs are easy to grow in your own kitchen! You don't need to have a "green thumb" or a huge garden to reap the benefits of these amazing herbs. But if you aren't able to have your own herb garden, buy organic herbs in bulk and store them in the freezer to have on hand at all times.

Fresh herbs like parsley, rosemary, oregano, and basil are the most nutritious plants you can consume. For example, everyone thinks spinach is the perfect food, but fresh oregano has eight times the amount of antioxidants! Sure, we don't eat a cup of oregano like we would spinach, but it does go to show that a little bit provides a huge benefit.

Instead of consuming fruits and starchy veggies that have fructose and raise blood sugar quickly, I suggest using herbs and spices, which often have many more vitamins, minerals and phytonutrients than any fruit will give you.

> **HEALTH TIP:** I suggest purchasing organic herbs. Unlike an avocado that has a thick protective shell that you discard, you eat the leaves that pesticides may have been sprayed on.

The chart below demonstrates how herbs are much better than fruits and vegetables as sources for vitamins and minerals:

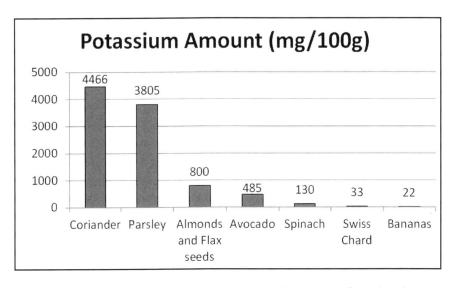

As you can see, there is more potassium in 1 tablespoon of parsley than in a whole banana, and it comes without all the inflammatory sugar.

SUMMARY

The take-home message is that fructose increases the rate of fat accumulation, blood pressure, triglycerides, insulin resistance, type 2 diabetes, and stimulates inflammation that activates the immune system. Strokes, coronary artery disease, heart disease, and aortic aneurysms are just a few of the complications linked to indulging in fructose.

Don't accept that a cookie or soft drink made with raw coconut sugar, agave nectar, or something else "natural" is healthy. I can't believe how many clients reach out to me stating they eat a "clean diet" and still feel terrible. When I dive into what they are eating, they tell me "Lara bars"... basically dried fruit and nuts. Yes, I suppose that could be considered a "clean diet," but why isn't it working? Albert Einstein's definition of insanity is to continue doing the same thing over and over again and expecting different results. Cut out the sugar! I feel that the words "organic date cookie" is an oxymoron. Your body doesn't care: sugar is sugar once it hits the bloodstream. Just because it's a cookie made with USDA-certified organic dates plowed under a Fair Trade banner, it is still sugar.

People often flip out when I tell them the only fruits they are ever allowed are avocados, olives, tomatoes, lemons, and limes. It's not a matter of being happy excluding all other fruits; it's about stepping outside of what you've been taught and seeing another way of doing things. If you have a "perfectly" operating metabolism, you're right, a couple of pieces of fruit "won't hurt you." But unfortunately, the majority of people (anyone with illness, inflammation, achy muscles or joints, digestive troubles, weight issues ... the list goes on) will do better with no sugar in their diet, not even from fruit. We are overloaded with fructose from many sources, and fructose is actually toxic to the liver — fructose is not metabolized the same way as glucose, its entire metabolic load rests on the liver. If you suffer with any kind of fatigue (such as CFS or adrenal fatigue) you will want to avoid all sources of fructose as well as sugar and grains in general. Really, we are meant to eat mostly veggies, since fruits are seasonal and not meant to be eaten all year long anyway. Our ancestors were eating in autumn to add fat for the long winter fast. So unless you are planning on fasting this winter, skip the fruit.

Chapter 5

Supplementing Keto-Adaptation

I am a health and wellness professional and am exposed to various diets and nutrition plans. Through my own research, personal trials or client experience, I have a strong understanding of how one can gain control of their weight and establish a healthy relationship with food. Of course, not one nutritional profile works for everyone and I highly advise individuals to do their own research and application to find what fits for their lifestyle and goals.

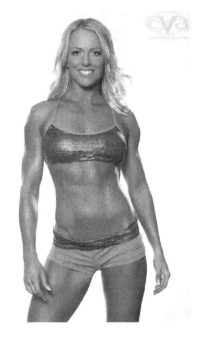

As a pro figure competitor, I have run the gamut when it comes to using nutrition in order to strip away body fat while preserving muscle mass. For many years, I followed the advice of most competition prep coaches—six to seven meals a day with a typical a mix of lean proteins, complex carbohydrates and healthy fats adding up to near 1800 calories. The first few times following this stringent clean eating plan, with an occasional 'cheat' meal, worked wonders as my body responded in the expected way. However, as I tried to maintain this lifestyle it became less and less effective. I always felt hungry and unsatisfied, I experienced cravings—mostly for sweets, and emotionally I wasn't feeling my best. Worst of all, I wasn't seeing the results I desired while preparing for another competition. I hit a plateau in my process that I couldn't seem to get around resulting in a disappointing finish on show day.

After struggling for a few more months trying to continue this way of eating, I began to pay more attention to what Maria Emmerich was posting on social media and then borrowed a few of her books from a friend. I was skeptical at first, thinking her method was very extreme, but realized I had nothing to lose at attempting ketosis. I transitioned away from my complex carbs (sweet potatoes, oatmeal, brown rice and quinoa) slowly, eliminating one serving at a time and introducing more fats (butter, coconut oil, etc.). Once the grains were completely eliminated, I began to notice a change. This change was not only physical but emotional. I felt more satisfaction with my meals, a reduction in cravings and overall balance with my mood.

My body responded in a way that was better than ever before. I never felt deprived throughout my most recent competition prep and did not follow a typical deplete the week before the show. My strength only continued to improve throughout the process, whereas in the past it always decreased during this process. After all other competitions, the following days or weeks are difficult finding a balance with 'treats' and 'normal' eating. This last time around, I felt a strong sense of control and minimal urge to stray from the Maria way. I was happy and knew that I had found something I could maintain, not only for show prep, but for life.

I still continue to model my nutrition after Maria's recommendations and have maintained my figure with more stability and less fluctuation. I don't often feel as though I am missing out on anything and know that including plenty of healthy fats in my diet, rather than a focus on complex carbs, has helped this change occur. I am able to maintain high energy and strength to fuel my day and my workouts using ketosis.

To me, after reading and researching Maria's ketosis method, it makes complete sense and will not be turning back!
—Sienna

A large piece of the weight-loss puzzle is cellular energy production. Many diet products contain stimulants, such as ephedra, which unnaturally stimulate thermogenesis (also known as the production of energy and heat).. These products may work for a while, but they leave you feeling tired and edgy when they wear off. On the other hand, amino acids, coenzyme Q10, and alpha-lipoic acid are some nutrients that are found in food that, in therapeutic doses, naturally optimize your body's cellular energy production. Not only do these nutrients provide greater energy and endurance and a greater ability to lose body fat, they help prevent aging in our cells. The food you eat and your exercise regime will work in combination with your cellular energy production to lead to either weight loss or weight gain. It is imperative for you to understand that what you eat is the most important factor. You can take all the cellular-enhancing supplements in the world, but if you are not changing your eating habits, you are wasting your money.

Many of you may be wondering, "Are these nutrients safe to take?" And yet, you won't think twice about popping an Advil because commercials claim it will take care of your "aches and pains." Advil, or ibuprofen, is a chemical that is foreign to our body, whereas the supplements I believe in are either found in food (only in concentrated, therapeutic doses) or found in our body (we just need more of it, like coenzyme Q10). In this chapter, I will discuss some top supplements that aid in a healthy keto-adapted journey. These supplements aren't a prerequisite for getting healthy, and I never thought supplements were necessary, but I am now a true believer; they have helped all of my clients heal so much faster.

When I work with clients, I often suggest a few key supplements to just about everyone: magnesium, potassium, salt, bone broth, bifido bacteria, a quality multivitamin, a quality omega-3, CoQ10, vitamin D (depending on your serum levels), and vitamin K. I'm an advocate in receiving most of your vitamins and minerals from foods, but since many clients do not eat liver or organ meat and forget to add herbs and spices into a daily routine, a multivitamin is just good insurance. If you do decide to add in a multi-vitamin, do not waste your money. Get a quality non-synthetic vitamin.

Bifidobacteria

Since I discussed magnesium and potassium in previous chapters, I want to start off with bifidobacteria, which I think is most important for everyone, babies included! A healthy body has about 2 pounds of good gut bacteria. Most of my clients and their children, however, are totally devoid of this healthy bacterium due to a lack of fermented vegetables in their diet and because they take antibiotics.

Anyone suffering from digestive problems, depression, yeast infections, chronic fatigue, allergies, IBS, or cravings should take supplemental bifido-bacteria daily. Eating fermented vegetables daily is a natural cure. Don't turn your nose up at the idea — they are really good! I have a recipe in chapter 10 that will give you a few ideas. As well, if you like a little spice, you must try kimchi!

> **HEALTH TIP:** Once your kimchi or fermented veggies are gone, drink the liquid they are stored in. I suggest at least ¼ cup of the fermented liquid about 15 minutes before meals to help with digestion, acid reflux and eliminate sugar cravings.

If you or your children have a history of using antibiotics, you must know that it causes your gut to be more susceptible for parasites and for candida overgrowth. A healthy large intestine is very acidic and has lots of beneficial bacteria such as Lactobacillus acidophilus. These healthy microorganisms feed on the waste left over from our digestion and create lactic acid. We need the lactic acid they produce in order to keep our colons healthy and in an acidic state. Without them, the colon does not have enough acidity to stop the growth of parasites and yeasts, and eventually the environment becomes hostile to acidophilus. (Remember that a healthy thyroid produces hydrochloric acid. If you have a damaged thyroid, supplementing with additional hydrochloric acid is a must)

> **HEALTH TIP:** Your gut contains 70% of your immune system. You can decrease the chance of food allergies in a fetus by taking bifidobacteria while pregnant.

Some of the signs of candida yeast overgrowth are fatigue, poor memory, a "spacey" feeling, intense food cravings, gas, loss of sexual desire, bad breath, and indigestion. Candida has also been directly linked to allergies, chronic fatigue syndrome, irritable bowel syndrome, multiple chemical sensitivity disorders, and various cancers. The use of antibiotics, birth control pills, alcohol, and refined foods all increase the risk of developing candida. The desired microorganisms that create lactic acid in the colon are naturally found in all vegetables and help turn cabbage into highly digestible sauerkraut. The fermentation process increases the amount of microorganisms.

Lactic acid also helps digestion at an earlier stage in our stomach. As we get older, our stomach's natural secretions of hydrochloric acid decrease. Hydrochloric acid breaks down food so it can be more easily absorbed by the small intestine. It is also the most important defense we have against harmful bacteria and parasites often present in food. Lactic acid can help compensate for reduced hydrochloric acid.

> **FUN FACT: Our moods are directly correlated to the intestinal flora of our gut; the nervous system actually comes from the gut to the brain. In the past, scientists thought the nervous system ran the other way. This is why what we put in our stomach is so essential to our mental health.**

Unpasteurized sauerkraut also benefits digestion in the stomach by assisting the pancreas. The pancreas secretes essential digestive enzymes into the stomach. Sauerkraut is high in enzymes that work just like the ones from the pancreas.

Having healthy intestinal flora, achieved with probiotics and fermented foods, increases our moods and decreases our cravings. When choosing a probiotic, always purchase the most effective strain of probiotics that creates an environment that yeasts cannot survive in. Probiotics in capsule form should always be stored in the fridge to prevent them from "dying" and becoming useless. These probiotics in capsule form can be purchased from most health food stores or the Internet, but remember that they must be kept cool; ensure the shipping time is not too long and that the storage facilities are adequate. Depending on your gut and immune health, dosage would be anywhere from one to three capsules of a quality probiotic that contains bifidobacteria about fifteen minutes to one hour before meals.

AMINO ACIDS

There are many different amino acids that come from protein. Since too much protein increases blood sugar, supplementing with specific amino acids instead can help in a variety of ways: tissue repair, healing leaky gut, muscle building, energy, as well as many other ailments. Different amino acids are responsible for different effects throughout our cells; some are more likely to contribute in glucogenesis, while others are very effective in increasing the rate of keto-adaptation.

1 L-LYCINE AND L-LEUCINE. Both lysine and leucine are amino acids that readily convert into ketone bodies. Lysine consumption ultimately harvests ketone bodies and acetoacetyl-CoA for use in energy production. Lysine helps your body produce carnitine, which is the next amino acid that I list in this chapter. According to the University of Maryland Medical Center, lysine also aids in calcium absorption and the construction of collagen, which is the protein that creates firm skin, healthy bones, cartilage, and tendons.

Leucine is one of the three essential amino acids that make up a branched-chain amino acid (BCAA); the other two acids are isoleucine and valine. L-leucine is the one I am mainly concerned with; it is known in the fitness community as the ultimate muscle builder and is crucial for attaining a positive nitrogen balance and for building lean muscle mass. It is referred to as an "essential" amino acid because your body cannot make it — you must get it through your diet. Unlike most amino acids, which are metabolized in the liver, BCAAs are metabolized in the muscles. They are fundamental for protein synthesis and for conserving muscle tissue. Leucine is an extra special amino acid because we need it to make use of all the other amino acids, such as L-glutamine and L-carnitine. Leucine produces acetyl-CoA and acetoacetate and is a ketogenic amino acid. Supplementing with leucine amino acids on a keto-adapted diet has permitted scientists to treat patients with epilepsy without having to resort to an excessively restrictive keto-adapted diet.

L-valine and L-isoleucine also make up BCAAs and they are helpful for other reasons. L-valine supports glucose metabolism and protein synthesis and boosts the immune system. It also aids in the detoxification of excess nitrogen in the liver. L-isoleucine aids in muscle recovery post-workout and is helpful in supporting blood sugar levels already within normal range. Isoleucine assists in hemoglobin formation and can increase energy levels and endurance in conjunction with a ketogenic diet.

Branched-chain amino acids have been demonstrated to increase recovery from a vegetative state in patients with traumatic brain injury. Studies on BCAA supplementation also show recovery of brain dopamine metabolism. The ailments that are relieved with BCAA supplementation are parallel to the benefits that have been shown to be aided by a well-formulated keto-adapted diet, a fact that is not a coincidence. One significant outcome of keto-adaptation that I mentioned in chapter 2 is an intense increase in the circulation of BCAAs in our body; this is because we are using fat as fuel instead of glucose. So as you start your well-formulated keto-adapted diet, there is less of a need for extra BCAAs. Adding in extra BCAAs to your keto-adapted journey will help you, but diet is first and foremost.

These amino acids, specifically L-leucine and L-lycine, are ketogenic amino acids; when taken together, they help to produce energy in your muscles, promote protein synthesis, and give you a little more forgiveness with your carbohydrate and protein intake. I suggest taking 1000 mg of L-lycine and 1500 mg of L-leucine in the morning.

2 L-CARNITINE. L-carnitine is an amino acid that aids the breakdown of fat by shuttling triglycerides into the mitochondria, our body's "fat-burning powerhouse." Discovered in 1905, it is a water-soluble, vitamin-like compound that is readily used in the body. Dietary carnitine can be found in a number of foods. The best source is meat, particularly beef, sheep, and lamb.

The American Chronicle also states there is another significant reason that makes carnitine stand out among the various other weight-loss supplements. Carnitine has the unique distinction of keeping watch and restricting the accumulation of fat around the liver and heart. This unique supplement also helps enhance muscle strength and aids in the reduction of triglyceride levels in the body. Carnitine also helps reduce irritability and anxiety, common side effects amongst dieters. This supplement can help increase your energy while simultaneously suppressing your appetite. Muscular fatigue is also reduced, which can help you go longer and harder in your fitness routine. I suggest taking 3 grams of L-carnitine in the morning.

3 L-GLUTAMINE. L-glutamine is a particularly important supplement for anyone wanting to lose weight. Glutamine is mainly stored within the muscles and is the body's most abundant amino acid. Amino acids are the basic building blocks of a protein. Glutamine is my favorite supplement and one that I take pretty much all the time. It is an amazing supplement that helps a variety of people: the dieter; the workout warrior; the chronically ill; people with stomach and intestinal issues, acid reflux, and leaky gut; cancer patients; and those recovering from surgery. All of the people described above should be taking glutamine regularly.

Glutamine is extra important to those who exercise. It is used up very quickly during prolonged and intense cardiovascular workouts, such as running and aerobics, and our body cannot make as much as it needs. This is bad because it causes the body to burn muscle for energy, exhausting our glutamine supply even further. Glutamine supplements enhance your body's ability to recover and to stay healthy. After intense exercise, your body's immune system is in a weakened condition, making you more vulnerable to infections and disease. Experts recommend taking glutamine supplements within five minutes after completing a workout or as soon as possible in order to give muscles the best chance of becoming the lean, mean, fat burning machines we want them to be.

Glutamine has three main factors that increase athletic performance. The first is its ability to rebuild muscle tissue. This doesn't directly make them bigger, but it allows for the muscles to recover faster, resulting in a better workout next time. The more you can continue to challenge your body with exercise, the better your results will be. The second factor is that glutamine supports our body's ability to reload our muscles with nutrients. This directly relates to your muscles' ability to increase lean body tissue, an act that raises our metabolism. The third important factor for athletes is that glutamine increases our human growth hormone output, also known as our fat-burning hormone.

Glutamine is also extremely helpful in the prevention of muscle breakdown caused by intense stress, physical injury, severe burns, disease, overexertion, poor nutrition, and dieting. Glutamine is extra special because it is the only amino acid that contains two nitrogen molecules. This additional molecule takes the nitrogen to where it is needed most. Nitrogen is one of the building blocks of muscle cells, and glutamine is the delivery system for getting the nitrogen to those cells. Glutamine can also transport excess nitrogen out of the body, which is important because nitrogen can act as a toxin. The most favorable condition for muscle growth is when glutamine is working appropriately and when nitrogen intake is greater than nitrogen output.

Being overweight and having a body in an inflammatory state makes glutamine supplementation even more important. When the body is inflamed, it breaks down the muscle tissue to get the extra glutamine it needs — this results in muscle loss. Getting extra glutamine allows the body to lose weight and retain muscle mass.

Glutamine is also very therapeutic for our digestive system. Intestinal health is important because it is the transport of fuel and nutrients. Glutamine is the fuel and nourishes the cells that line the digestive track and intestines. Time and time again, studies have shown that a therapeutic dose of supplemental glutamine protects against aspirin-induced gastric lesions and helps heal painful ulcers. In fact, an old folk remedy for ulcers is cabbage juice, which is very high in glutamine. Stomach problems such as colitis and Crohn's disease can be calmed by glutamine. In fact, glutamine can be used whenever there are any stomach problems, from something as simple as drinking too much alcohol (alcoholic-induced gastritis) to ulcers, diarrhea, or even more serious problems such as inflammatory bowel disease.

More Benefits of Glutamine

Glutamine is also beneficial for a variety of other health issues.

1. Studies find that glutamine will reduce cravings for high-glycemic carbohydrates and can make your weight-loss plan a lot easier.

2. Glutamine can help prevent both depression and fatigue and can also help us create neurotransmitters in the brain, which help relax us while elevating our mood. In the brain, glutamine is transformed into glutamic acid and boosts the amount of GABA (gamma-aminobutyric acid). Both glutamic acid and GABA are considered "brain fuel" because they are necessary for everyday mental function.

3. Many studies have found that therapeutic amounts of glutamine help prevent the harmful effects of alcohol on the brain and may also decrease alcohol (as well as sugar) cravings.

4. Glutamine is essential to our immune system because it is utilized by white blood cells. It is now used in some hospitals intravenously to speed up recovery of patients. The better you develop your muscles through exercise, the more glutamine they will produce, which is one of the reasons fit people get sick less often.

A recent study published by The American Journal of Clinical Nutrition has shown that oral supplementation with as little as 2 grams of glutamine significantly enhanced patients' overall health!

Glutamine is considered a safe substance. Dosages of up to 21 grams a day have been demonstrated to have no negative side effects. High glutamine levels also support brain function, including better alertness. Taking 2 grams before bed increases our human growth hormone. The recommended dosage is 5 to 20 grams a day for optimal health. I prefer clients take 2 to 3 grams (depending on gut health) about fifteen to thirty minutes before meals. It can be taken with food, but it really helps to deter cravings if taken before meals.

Alpha Lipoic Acid (ALA)

Alpha lipoic acid is an amazing supplement for a variety of reasons. It is a powerful antioxidant and anti-inflammatory and is both water- and fat-soluble. Because alpha lipoic acid is found only in trace amounts in food, it must be taken as a supplement. Alpha lipoic acid is found naturally in the body, inside the mitochondria. It is closely involved in the energy production of the cell. Alpha lipoic acid, like many other nutrients (including L-carnitine and CoQ10), enhances our ability to metabolize food into energy.

Do you complain of sagging skin or cellulite? A high-carbohydrate diet causes a natural process called glycation, in which the sugar in your bloodstream attaches to proteins to form harmful new molecules called advanced glycation end products, or AGEs (as discussed in chapter 3). The more carbohydrates you eat, the more AGEs you develop. As AGEs accumulate, they damage neighboring proteins in a domino-like manner. Collagen and elastin, the protein fibers that keep skin firm and elastic, are most vulnerable when you are eating a high-starch diet. Once the damage has been done, the supple and strong collagen and elastin become dry and delicate, leading to wrinkles and sagging. AGEs deactivate your body's natural antioxidant enzymes, leaving you more vulnerable to sun damage. Adding in 600 mg of alpha lipoic acid (ALA) can help repair the skin from your past years of being a sugar burner. If you are going to spend the money on ALA supplements and serums, make sure to get them from a quality source from Germany. Chinese ALA is processed with harsh and toxic chemicals.

ALA is both fat- and water-soluble, so it helps decrease inflammation pretty much throughout the whole body. It safeguards our fatty membranes and it helps our cells with controlling blood sugar, which in turn helps the process of keto-adaptation along. Blood glucose levels and insulin sensitivity are much improved when you supplement with quality ALA. This insulin-sensitizing effect is also seen in L-carnitine and other supplements discussed in this chapter. An increase in insulin sensitivity helps slow aging and speeds up the recovery process. ALA is a great supplement for anyone dealing with diabetes. Some other cool facts on ALA:

1. Alpha lipoic acid acts as a coenzyme in the production of energy by converting carbohydrates into energy. Athletes may recognize this as ATP.

2. ALA is the only antioxidant that can enhance levels of glutathione, our most important antioxidant to health and youth.

I usually recommend 600 mg of ALA at breakfast for clients starting a keto-adapted diet. If you purchase the newer version of ALA called r-alpha lipoic acid, you only need 200 mg daily; it is more potent and much more expensive. Don't take it too late in the day since it is energizing.

CoQ10

Coenzyme Q10 is an antioxidant nutrient found in each and every cell of the body. This antioxidant helps the body produce energy within each cell. We know that mitochondria generate cellular energy; it is also where fat-burning takes place. The more CoQ10 we have, the more mitochondria are created; therefore, more fat-burning. Working together with the other metabolic supplements (such as L-carnitine, green tea, and alpha-lipoic acid), CoQ10 increases metabolism, providing greater energy, endurance, and ability to lose body fat, while also preventing the energy decline seen in aging cells. It also assists in weight loss by regulating blood sugar, enhancing insulin sensitivity, and maximizing the movement of fats in our blood to be used for fuel.

Hundreds of studies document the effectiveness of CoQ10 in protecting all vital organs of the body, including the brain, heart, and kidneys. Because of its powerful anti-inflammatory effects, CoQ10 is extremely protective of the cardiovascular system. It keeps the heart muscle healthy and also prevents inflammation in the arteries (which can lead to arteriosclerosis). The ability of coenzyme Q10 to effectively pump blood to your heart leaves you with immense energy. Also, the viscosity of blood is lowered, which makes the heart function more efficiently.

Coenzyme Q10 also boosts your immune system. The ability of your body to deal with diseases increases because the level of antibodies also increases. This important nutrient prevents gum diseases as well by enabling the healing power of your gums, thus giving them greater strength. Coenzyme Q10 is very helpful for weight loss, multiple sclerosis, high blood pressure, diabetes, chronic fatigue, muscle weakness, and muscular dystrophy.

Adam Russell, PhD, a human-performance expert, has stated that "long-term CoQ10 supplementation may help athletes to recover more quickly after high-intensity workouts." A 2008 study published in the *Journal of the International Society of Sports Nutrition* reported that fourteen days of CoQ10 increased trained athletes' time to exhaustion in an endurance exercise test.

Although CoQ10 can be found in small amounts in fish, such as sardines or salmon, as well as in nuts, supplementation is best for anti-aging and for weight loss. CoQ10 supplementation is of particular importance for females because women tend to have lower levels than men.

This nutrient is something I recommend for everyone, especially for clients who have been on statins. Statin drugs inhibit the body's synthesis of this significant nutrient, a process that causes people to be lower in energy because it depletes their mitochondria health.

People mistakenly think that they need to exercise to create a calorie deficit in order to lose weight. This is not how exercise helps with weight loss. Exercise builds muscle and muscle builds mitochondria. It is in the mitochondria where fat is oxidized so you can keep your cells and liver insulin-sensitized. Weight loss and energy are directly correlated to the health of your mitochondria. You can increase mitochondria with fasting, with exercise, and with adding in CoQ10. The increase in mitochondria increases circulation; it helps eliminate migraines, headaches, numbness, and tingling. I recommend taking 400 mg of CoQ10 at breakfast.

Summary

The noteworthy message I want to leave you with is that a well-formulated keto-adapted diet achieves by itself what people hope to achieve by ingesting expensive supplements. A ketogenic diet will advance muscle growth and speed recovery to a much greater degree compared to a high-carbohydrate diet. If you have the desire to speed up your keto-adaptation process, however, supplements are shown to help.

Disclaimer: Always check with your primary health care professional before starting any supplement regime.

Chapter 6

Exercise and Performance

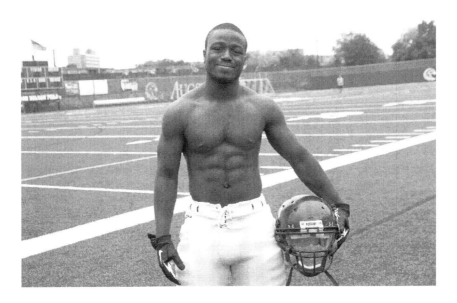

Growing up as a kid, I didn't even realize that my food options were actually going to help me out one day. What can I say, I am a "meat eater." I always got a lot of flack about not eating the bun or fries that came with my meal, but I just didn't have the taste buds for that stuff. I just craved meat, especially meats fried in good oils. I wasn't aware that my diet options would eventually affect my athleticism and structure as I got older and that I needed to be more aware of those things while in sports. I have eaten this way my whole life, but I feel so good when eating this way. It has helped my energy level and has also helped me "beef up" while going through high school and now into my college football career. We are put on a weight-lifting routine, and this diet has helped me to reach my goals and become in the best shape ever. And secondly, I do not drink. Hard to believe, I know. As a college student you would think I would be doing the partying and drinking. But I don't consume alcohol in any form due to the detrimental effects it has on everything that I am trying to achieve. I feel like I am in the best shape of my life and full of energy, and it's due mostly to my food choices, a low carb, high fat diet, and no alcohol intake. These things along with my weight program make me feel stronger than ever and able to achieve my goals.

—Ericson

As I stated at the end of the last chapter, many people mistakenly think that they need to exercise to create a calorie deficit in order to lose weight, but this is not how exercise helps with weight loss. Exercise builds muscle and muscle builds mitochondria. It is in the mitochondria where fat is oxidized so you can keep your cells and liver insulin sensitized. Even personal trainers misguidedly believe that exercise is about the calorie expenditure. It is actually about hormones, specifically insulin.

My love for movement and exercise did *not* come easily for me. Sure, I liked to play as a kid, but when it came to phys-ed, let's just say I wasn't the first kid picked to be on any team. You wouldn't have guessed that now, based on my activity level. The reason I want you to really soak this in is because even if you are about to skip this chapter because you don't think you will ever be an active person, think again!

I still remember when I was in middle school, pacing back and forth in my parents' yard and contemplating how to get out of the dreaded "mile run" that I had to do in phys-ed the next day. My anxiety about this was getting the best of me. I remember thinking how I could break my leg so I didn't have to run, because if I were just to say that I was sick that day, the teacher would just make me run it the next week. I had to think of something more long term. Not wanting to actually break my leg, how could I fake a broken leg? All of these ridiculous ideas went through my head!

If I told you that now, at age 33, I run every morning because I love it (not because of weight loss), would you believe me? It's true. I run every morning and it isn't because I'm training for a race or because I'm trying to lose weight. I do it because I love it. It is my quiet time that I adore.

You may be thinking, "I will never be a morning person that will get up early to exercise." When I say I run in the morning, don't mistake me and think that I do it first thing. I don't. Sure, I am lucky with the fact that I don't have to drive to an office to work. You may not think that my exercise schedule is practical, but I want you to see how I include intermittent fasting into my exercise schedule. You could still try it on the weekends or on your days off work. You don't have to do this daily like I do.

I have always been a morning person — I get up at about 5:30 a.m. so I have no distractions with work. I either have early morning client appointments, email clients, or I work on writing recipes and my blog for about two to two and a half hours. Then I put on my running shoes and run for about an hour. Then I have breakfast. While I work on the computer, I have hot tea or a very hot decaf Americano. I also take amino acids when I wake up, but other than that, no food. I find that I focus better while I fast. This is easy for me now, but it wasn't always. I also wasn't always able to go this long before eating, but as work increased, I unintentionally kept increasing the time in my morning fast and it got easier as time went on.

I also don't stop there when it comes to movement. I think I'm a little addicted; I feel like the "Energizer Bunny" on this diet, and I no longer have an afternoon crash. I also love yoga, riding my bike, kayaking, swimming, you name it! You can often catch me walking and answering emails. I hate sitting at my computer. My energy is through the roof because I have a lot of healthy mitochondria in my cells.

Three days a week on my lunch break, I lift weights. And not pink dumbbells. I lift heavy weights, really heavy weights. I love it when a new guy comes to the weight lifting class that I take (called BodyPump) and tries to squat as much as me, determined to make sure he lifts more than any girl in class. But at the end of the six minutes of squats, he finally turns to talk to me afterwards, saying, "Wow, you are really strong." If you are unfamiliar with BodyPump, it is a class where you lift weights to tracks. Each track is about four to six minutes long. You start out with a warm-up, then listen to a song for squats, chest, back, triceps, biceps, lunges, shoulders, and abs, and then have a cool down. The whole class is a little less than an hour, and when I added this into my life, wow … my body changed!

With that said, do not think that you need to workout and move non-stop in order to lose weight. I have many clients who do little to no exercise and still look amazing on a keto-adapted diet. The purpose of me describing to you my activity level is to show how much energy I have now that I have lots of healthy mitochondria and to also show that you do not need to add in carbohydrates if you start to exercise.

Take Chad, for example. He does about fifteen minutes of band-resistant training five days a week in the winter months. He only does it in the winter because he is very busy with work in the summer.

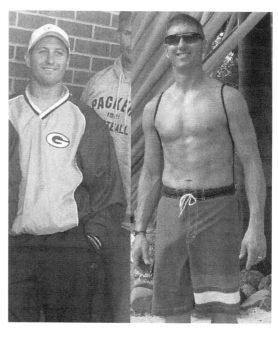

I have never been what I would consider overweight. I've always been in very good shape, very active and thought I looked pretty good for an "old guy" :) A few years ago, my wife's friend Maria opened our eyes to a lot of our food choices. We took baby steps and it's still a learning process, but we have turned over to a grain-free, low-carb, high-fat diet, and I can't believe the difference in my body composition. Of course I didn't change anything except for my diet, and I lost sixteen pounds and look way leaner than before without having to even lift hard! My workout routine is very limited and for a limited amount of the year. I only have time in the few winter months of November through March to workout, and my workout routine is strictly using the resistance bands and some calisthenics which include push-ups, pull-ups and a few other things. I was amazed at how effective it was and am completely sold on the eating plan! I am definitely enjoying my food choices as well. What guy doesn't love that diet ... I love my food and never feel hungry. I am in the best shape of my life and feel great. It's made a huge difference in keeping up with my kids and playing sports, as I am still very active in sports. I can see for sure that it's not just all exercise, but a huge part is the diet and food options. :)

—Chad O.

HEALTH TIP: SLEEP IN OR EXERCISE? I love that Chad shared his before-and-after photo because he looks amazing with little exercise and eating a well-formulated keto-adapted diet. I want to stress that waking up early and skimping on sleep is not what I would prefer clients to do. Sleep trumps exercise in my opinion. When you get quality sleep, all of your hormones are balanced. If you wake up at 5 a.m. to get a workout in to help with calorie expenditure, you are actually shooting yourself in the foot. Without adequate amounts of sleep, you stimulate leptin and ghrelin which cause increased hunger and a deminished ability to feel "full" even with sufficient amounts of food. People who are night owls and are nighttime eaters also have higher RQs and low fat oxidation rates. Get to bed people!

There is a phenomenon called sarcopenia, where we lose 1% of muscle a year starting at age 25. I suggest you add in weight training yesterday! OK, start tomorrow. In order to slow the loss of muscle, you must give up carbohydrates. By switching to be a ketone burner, aside from using fats for energy, you are helping prevent muscle loss since the need for glucose is reduced. Muscle tissue breakdown occurs when there is a need for an amount of glucose that exceeds the stores of glycogen. Fasting will also prevent muscle loss. The dominant hormones in a fasted state (human growth hormone, glucagon, and adrenaline) are responsible for catabolizing tissue and can aid in the breakdown of fats from the glycerol backbone. They also use fats for oxidation for energy instead of sugar. To read more on intermittent fasting, check out chapter 9 on Helpful Tips.

HEALTH TIP: Alcohol decreases your testosterone levels and increases bad estrogen by up to 300 percent for up to 24 hours after you finish drinking.

I just wanted to send you a quick note to tell you how much your nutrition and exercise philosophy has changed the way I approach a healthy lifestyle. When I first picked up your book Secrets to a Healthy Metabolism *a few years ago, I was strictly a long distance runner who fueled those runs with a lot of pasta and pancakes! What I struggled with on a daily basis was intense cravings for sugar — it was miserable! While reading your book, everything started to click — I was craving sugar because I was feeding my body sugar around the clock! I soon began to turn my nutrition around. I traded out pancakes for eggs, sausage, and veggies, and [traded] pasta for salads loaded with veggies, chicken, and healthy fats. I can now say that I live craving free ... I never thought that was possible!*

I was also stunned when I read in your book that exercise does not equal weight loss. What? I felt that all my years of running was a waste of time! I started to incorporate weightlifting and HIIT training. The combination of these exercises along with proper nutrition started to bring about change in my body composition that running on a high-sugar diet never did. I still do some longer runs, but I do them because I enjoy them! Thank you for giving me the gift of fantastic health and freedom Maria! Keep up all the great work you do! You touch so many lives!
—Nicole

As I work with clients, I meet people with a variety of lifestyles. Some clients prefer not to exercise, which is just fine, and they do wonderful on the diet (proof that weight loss is 80% diet). Then there is the other extreme, where I get clients who are training for a marathon and are wanting to increase carbs now because they need to "carb load." I often get asked, "My son is in high school football; if you don't recommend Gatorade, what should he drink?" How about water? There is a much better way to fuel our bodies for performance than carbs.

Myth: You need carbohydrates to fuel exercise

Facts:

1. Our bodies store over 40,000 calories of fat, but we can only store 2,000 calories of carbs. This is why, when "carb-burning," marathoners "hit-the-wall" and constantly need gel packs and Gatorade. They are

still low in performance at the end of races, too, due to the depletion of carbs in their muscles and liver.

2. Carb-fueling tactics and sugar-based fuel sources create a body that fuels on carbs while simultaneously inhibits fat burning. Dr. Volek and Dr. Phinney state in *The Art and Science of Low Carbohydrate Performance*, "This suppression of fat burning lasts for days after carbs are consumed, not just the few hours following their digestion."[47]

3. Even athletes who have very little body fat are able to work out twenty times longer at their max level. Vigorous exercise fueled on carbs depletes the athlete in a few hours, but by burning fat for fuel, you can exercise for days.

> **HEALTH TIP:** Fat release plummets with a moderate increase in insulin. This is why I am so extreme; even a banana will cause fat burning to stop, and you are no longer "keto-adapted." Is a banana the "devil"? No, but for what we want to accomplish, it is going to stop your efforts.

Any person training for a marathon or endurance race must read Dr. Volek and Dr. Phinney's book *The Art and Science of Low Carbohydrate Performance*. But if the idea of running until your big toe nail falls off (which mine did on my first marathon) doesn't appeal to you, check out Dr. Volek's other book, *The Art and Science of Low Carbohydrate Living*, which is for everyone, not just athletes.

It is especially interesting when Dr. Volek points out that he thought with all the data in the studies they conducted (he and Dr. Phinney have over sixty years of research combined) and with low-carb approaches, he thought they would change the world of performance. Yet, we have been so brainwashed that these studies came out with a thud. (Not to mention our government-driven, high-carb food industry doesn't want you to know this.) The idea that you can run marathons on ketones (which is what I do) is still considered crazy! It does take a few weeks to become "keto-adapted" with a very low-carbohydrate approach, but if you give it time, I promise you, your energy will be "through the roof"!

> **HEALTH TIP:** The heart muscle prefers ketones, and the brain runs optimally on ketones with minimal glucose. Our entire existence as a species has relied on this evolutionary adaptation. Entire civilizations existed for centuries on what is essentially a zero-carb diet. There is no genuine necessity for any "essential carbohydrates" in our diet. You can live a very healthy and long life never consuming carbohydrates, as long as you get adequate quality protein and fat. What is so interesting is that if you flip this, the same cannot be said. Without protein or fat, you eventually get depression, thyroid disorders, Alzheimer's ... shall I go on? If you cut back too much on protein or fat you will ultimately get sick and die.

Benefits of a Keto-Adapted Diet When Exercising

1. It improves insulin sensitivity and speeds recovery time between training sessions. Low-carb diets are anti-inflammatory. This produces less oxidative stress while exercising, which speeds recovery time between exercise sessions. This is why I was able to run every day while training for my marathons.

2. It spares protein from being oxidized, which preserves muscle. Branched-chain amino acids are considered essential because your body can't make them, so you need to consume them for proper muscle building and repair (as well replenishing red blood cells). What I found so interesting is that BCAA oxidation rates usually rise with exercise, which means you need more if you are an athlete. But in keto-adapted athletes, ketones are burned in place of BCAA. Critics of low-carb diets claim that you *need* insulin to grow muscles; however, in a well-designed low-carb, high-fat diet there is less protein oxidation and double the amount of fat oxidation, which leaves your muscles in place while all you burn is fat!

Jimmy Moore from Livin' La Vida Low-Carb did an experiment while he was (and still is) on a keto-adapted diet. Jimmy writes, "When I was in the midst of my own personal n=1 experiment of nutritional ketosis in 2012, I decided to see what was happening to my body fat loss and muscle mass growth using a DXA scan. I had one done in September 2012, started a 20-minute slow lifting program every three days, and then got another DXA again two months later in November 2013 to see what changes would take place. I was stunned to find that I not only lost over 16 pounds of body fat but I also simultaneously gained over 6 pounds of muscle! I'll be sharing much more about the power of a high-fat, low-carb ketogenic approach on so many aspects of health in my book *Keto Clarity* coming in June 2014.*"

3. It decreases the build up of lactate, and therefore helps control pH and respiratory function. A myth of low-carb diets is that it puts you in a state of acidosis.

   Dr. Volek and Dr. Phinney point out that "This stems from the unfortunate fact that many doctors confuse nutritional ketosis (blood ketones at 1-3 millimolar) with keto-acidosis (blood ketones greater than 20 millimolar). In nutritional ketosis, blood pH at rest stays normal, plus sharp drops in pH due to CO_2 and lactate buildup during exercise are restrained. By contrast, in keto-acidosis, blood pH is driven abnormally low by the 10-fold greater buildup of ketones. Suggesting these 2 states are similar is like equating a gentle rain with a flood because they both involve water."

4. It improves cognition. Ketones aren't just fuel for our body, but they are also great for our brain. They provide substrates to help repair damaged neurons and membranes. This is why I really push a high-fat, low-carb diet for clients who suffer from Alzheimer's (type 3 diabetes) and seizures.

5. It doesn't damage our immune system and produces less free radical damage to our cells.

Exercise and Stress on the Body

I love exercise for so many reasons. For me, it boosts my soul and makes me happy. I love my morning run in the country: seeing deer, the silence, the feeling of gratitude that fills me ... It took me years to enjoy running.

When I first started, I remember aiming for half a mile, and that was tough. Now I run every morning without hardship, and I do it because I love it, not for weight loss.

I did however sign up for a marathon six years ago for weight loss, and guess what happened? I *gained* weight. Yes, I did go a little over-board with my training — I am a type A personality. I was running two times a day. I would get on the scale and it would go up! Argh!. I ate the same low carb way … what was going on? I was over-training, I went beyond excessive cardio. My high-intensity exercise routine pushed my body's stress response too far, which lead to a cascade of biochemical responses that could have caused damage to my health.

First, let's be more specific. Most people do cardio to lose weight, though some people are more focused on the number on the scale rather than "fat" loss. The majority of "fat" in our body (over 80%) is collected in one form and is stored in our body's fat cells. To get rid of fat, we can use it as energy, which is a process called lipolysis. But if you are a sugar burner, meaning you fuel your body with carbs before you exercise, you don't initiate the human growth hormone to burn fat. Instead, you just burn sugar.

> **RACING TIP:** What really gets to me is how people serve bread, bananas, and chips at the end of a marathon! My husband Craig would always have to pack a cooler with my recovery food, which made it difficult to find him in the crowds. I also packed my amino acids in my pocket so I could at least speed my recovery along with those. The amino acids from protein are what repair our cells, not actual protein. I suggest packing your own "recovery" meal and extra amino acids for proper muscle recovery.

Too much cardio stimulates a stress hormone called cortisol. You have probably heard advertisements for weight loss drugs that reduce cortisol, the undesired "belly fat"-increasing hormone. Don't waste your money on these products. The easiest (and free) way to lower cortisol is to sleep! This is why most people gain weight in the summer —they don't get enough sleep.

Cortisol is the hormone that is released when the body is under stress. This stress can be from work, family, not enough sleep, bad eating habits, or excess exercise (such as marathon training); these stressors all stimulate cortisol. All of our hormones come in waves, like the ocean: cortisol is naturally high in the morning, but chronically high levels of cortisol increase your risk for a variety of health issues, including depression, weight gain, sleep disturbances, and digestive issues. Also, cortisol and testosterone seem to conflict. Aerobic work = more cortisol release = less available testosterone (and you know what that does) while cortisol is elevated.

Excess cardio also affects our brain neurotransmitters (such as serotonin, GABA, and dopamine) which are our feel-good, anti-anxiety brain waves. Cravings for carbohydrates and binge eating are associated with low serotonin levels. When you burn these out with stress and intense exercise, it leads to feelings of depression, chronic fatigue, and sleep disorders. A shortage of these healthy neurotransmitters negatively affect the hypothalamic-pituitary axis, which can cause serious conditions such as hypothyroidism.

> **HEALTH TIP:** A ketogenic diet increases the enthusiastic output of our mitochondria, reduces the production of damaging free radicals, and favors the production of GABA. GABA is a calming neurotransmitter that has a relaxing effect and is produced by ketosis. Ketosis alleviates pain and has an overall anti-inflammatory effect.[50]

This is why I ask my clients if their thyroid disorder appeared during a stressful event. Stress = excessive adrenal hormone output = adrenal burnout = adrenals steal from thyroid. Hypothyroidism is known to cause weight gain, depression, constipation, and digestive dysfunction along with other undesired problems. Again, stress can be from a loss of a loved one, family stress, work stress, exercise-induced stress, not enough sleep, and poor eating habits.

Excessively intense exercise can cause a variety of health problems, especially for those dealing with other concurrent stressors such as autoimmune disease, leaky gut, or adrenal fatigue. On the other hand, short, high-intensity workouts are awesome for stimulating the human growth hormone, which induces fat loss.

> **NUTRIENT TIMING TIP:** The best time to burn fat is when performing aerobic exercise first thing in the morning on an empty stomach and after drinking a large glass of water, or a little coffee, in order to avoid dehydration. You burn 300% more body fat in the morning on an empty stomach than at any other time in the day because your body does not have any glycogen or stored carbohydrates/sugar in the liver to burn. When this happens, your body has to go directly into the fat stores in order to get the energy necessary to complete the activity. You also increase your human growth hormone levels, which is the fat-burning hormone. The human growth hormone and insulin counteract each other. If one is high, the other is low — like a see-saw. So if you eat something, especially carbohydrates, before a workout, you will be spiking your insulin levels, meaning your growth hormone levels will be low.

I'm not against aerobic exercise, I just suggest a more moderate approach and view it as movement that you perform in your daily life. This way you stop thinking of exercise as a "chore" and see it more as a "hobby." If you view exercise as an enjoyable activity, it can:

FIGHT DEPRESSION. About 80% of my clients have either low moods or full blown depression. Why is this happening? I believe it is mainly the low-fat diets ruining our brain's communication, but I also think that we have become a society where we sit in our cars to commute to a job where we sit inside staring at a computer screen all day, only to then sit in our car to drive home. And maybe in the summer, you are home early enough to enjoy a bit of sunlight before night. This is a formula for depression. In our ancestors' Paleo days, we had hard jobs, but they were outside and we were active. My husband, Craig, traveled for work to Amsterdam. He was astonished how the people there rode bikes to work and that many of them had over twenty-five miles to commute! When Craig and I started to ride our bikes together, I felt like a little kid again. A smile immediately formed on my face as I felt the breeze on my face. We need to move more, preferably outside! Exercise cranks up the body's production of serotonin and dopamine, brain chemicals that are fundamental to a happy mood. It also boosts levels of the feel-good chemicals called endorphins.

GROW NEW BRAIN CELLS. Much like how plant food makes plants grow better and quicker, the chemical known as brain-derived neurotrophic factor (BDNF) fuels the development and proliferation of brain cells. The part of the brain responsible for memory is the hippocampus. The hippocampus is particularly vulnerable to age-related decline. The more you exercise, the more BDNF you produce. Neuroscientists at Cambridge University have revealed that aerobic exercise, specifically running, stimulates the brain to grow new gray matter, which has a huge impact on mental ability.[49] Cardio boosts blood flow to the brain, which delivers much-needed oxygen (the brain soaks up 20 percent of all the oxygen in your body).

LOWER SUGAR IN YOUR BLOOD. When you eat carbs or excess protein, your body turns it into glucose. In order for glucose to enter cells, it must be escorted by the hormone insulin. Unfortunately, overconsumption of carbohydrates causes the cells to become resistant to insulin. The body then has to pump out more and more of it, and blood sugar levels rise, often resulting in type 2 diabetes. And even if you don't develop type 2 diabetes, insulin resistance is bad for your brain. When brain cells are flooded by glucose, it adversely affects memory and causes "brain fog." Regular exercise can help reverse insulin resistance. Exercise increases insulin sensitivity, which stabilizes your blood sugar after you eat. The better your blood-sugar control, the more protected you are against age-related cognitive decline.

A Better Plan: Interval and Strength Training Combined

Many clients come to me being "cardio queens" in efforts to lose weight. In weight loss situations, I often steer them to my high-intensity strength training plan to get the after-burn effect and muscle gain. Your body will burn more calories after exercise when you use intervals (alternating between low- and high-intensity exercise) than it does after you do slow, consistent cardio, and your metabolism will stay high. This is referred to this as the "after-burn" effect. Within a short time frame, the intervals, combined with strength training, make your muscles go crazy with activity; I call this a metabolic disturbance. This crazy metabolism boost causes lots of calorie burning after exercise to get your body back to normal. The result is you end up burning more fat and more calories in the post-exercise period as your body tries to get things under control.

WHY HIGH-INTENSITY STRENGTH TRAINING IS AWESOME:

1. It saves time. If you normally spend an hour and a half in the gym following the "fat burning zone" philosophy, you'll work yourself just as hard in forty-five minutes with high-intensity strength training.

2. Higher intensities stimulate your mitochondria growth.

3. It increases metabolism far more after the workouts than lower intensity training does. This means you continue to burn calories and fat for long periods after you're done training. Not so with the "fat burning zone." This "after-burn" effect can burn an extra 150-250 calories after you stop exercising.

4. It combats boredom. It's fun, and the time flies by during each session because you're working in cycles of high- and low-intensity work, instead of spending a long period of time at any one activity. I like to make a playlist of songs to match my intensity of the workout; a warm-

up song and a fast-paced song, followed by a slower-paced, recovery song where I lift weights, and repeat!

My plan of high-intensity strength training is based on a very simple concept: go fast, then lift weights as you catch your breath. Repeat. It sounds simple, but this formula has an incredible number of potential variations and strategies. To begin, start your workout at an easy pace and slowly increase your heart rate for at least five minutes. You can monitor this by using a heart rate monitor or by using a "rate of perceived exertion" test, a test that judges how hard your workout is by a rate of 1-10 (1 is resting, 10 is hardest possible workout). When you're warmed up, you're ready for an explosion of high-intensity work. Break into a jog or a sprint, depending on what "high intensity" means to you; your "rate of perceived exertion" should be around 8, and you shouldn't be able to carry on a conversation.

During the high-intensity periods, you're diminishing your body's ability to swap oxygen and carbon dioxide. You begin to feel the "burn" as your body eliminates lactic acid and your muscles start to lose their ability to contract. You are working so hard, you aren't physically able to continue this level of intensity for long. After a few minutes, stop your aerobic exercise, grab some free weights, and perform strength training exercises. Start with biceps and triceps. This period is called the "active recovery period."

Once you are finished with the biceps and triceps, get that heart rate back up by running as hard as you can. After a few minutes, grab the weights again, and move onto other body parts. Repeat this process for at least thirty minutes.

My exercise plan increases weight loss faster in many ways. Most importantly, it challenges your aerobic and anaerobic systems at the same time; in doing so, you're improving your body's mitochondria production and therefore your body's capacity to burn calories at a higher rate. You're also adding new muscle, which has lots of mitochondria. This helps speeds up your metabolism of fat even while at rest.

Interval training is effective at pushing you past plateaus in weight loss. Your body becomes a valuable fat-burning machine with all the healthy mitochondria. The mitochondrion is the only place in a cell where fat is burned and oxidized. It is the cell's "fat burning furnace."

> **NUTRIENT TIMING TIP:** Recent studies show that holding off and not eating for thirty minutes will increase human growth hormone (fat burning hormone) and will increase the "after-burn" effect even more. Remember the "after-burn" can help us burn an extra 150-250 calories after our workout while at rest! When you push your muscles to the point of exhaustion, it takes a lot of effort to repair them.

The exercise "after-burn" is the number of calories expended above resting values after a workout. Although intensity dependent, both aerobic and resistance training programs may elicit 150-250 (primarily fat) calories post workout. One pound of fat is equal to 3,500 calories. If you exercise five days a week, over the course of a year the "after-burn" would be calculated as follows: 5 workouts per week * 52 weeks * 100 EPOC calories / workout total 26,000 calories or 7 pounds of fat (The "after-burn" minimum is 100 calories, but if you can work harder and reach 250 calories … awesome.) Now, that's meaningful!

Workout Example

The following is an example of a good workout schedule:

WAKE UP (AFTER 8 HOURS OF RESTED SLEEP)

- Take the recommended morning supplements (including amino acid supplements) with 24 oz of water (green tea is best).

EXERCISE:

Workout on an empty stomach.
- Warm-Up for 5 minutes, then jog for 5 minutes
  - Do 10 push-ups, then 10 sit-ups
  - 9 push-ups, 9 sit-ups
  - 8 push-ups, 8 sit-ups
  - Repeat with 7, 6, 5, etc. all the way down to 1 push-up and 1 sit-up
- Jog for another 5 minutes
  - Do 10 triceps dips, then 10 bicep curls
  - 9 triceps dips, 9 bicep curls
  - Repeat with 8, 7, 6, etc. all the way down to 1 tricep dip and 1 bicep curl
- Jog for another 5 minutes
  - Do 10 squats (Advanced: hold weights in each hand), then 10 jumping jacks
  - 9 squats, 9 jumping jacks
  - Repeat with 8, 7, 6, etc. all the way down to 1 squat and 1 jumping jack (Repeat whole cycle if you are advanced)
- WALK for a cool down and stretch! Supplement with branch chain amino acids if desired.

15 MINUTES TO 1 HOUR BEFORE BREAKFAST:

- Take 2 grams of L-glutamine and one capsule of probiotics with bi-fidobacteria.

Summary

You can wipe out an entire workout's benefits in less than a minute simply by eating garbage. Without some structure and discipline to your nutrition, there is nothing that even my programs can do to help you lose fat. So make sure to include nutrition and interval training. These are the two mitochondria-building methods that will help you lose fat and get lean. Even if you just completed the above workout, put down the pasta, the breads, and the rice and step away from the table.

Chapter 7

How Keto-Adaption Heals Autoimmune Disorders

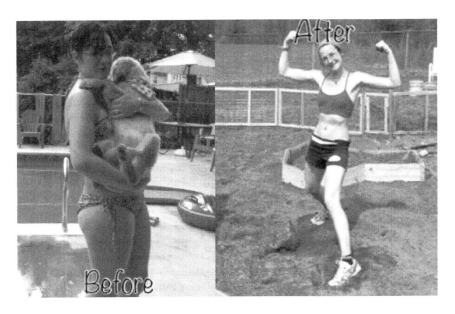

Before after severe soy allergy discovery, and eating locally and real food. The picture doesn't show all the gastrointestinal pain and general icky feelings that disappeared as well! —Cooper

For many years, I have been plagued with many autoimmune maladies. Most of them were just bothers like skin problems, aches, and burning tongue. I had been on a low dose of prednisone since 2002. About a year and a half ago, I was diagnosed with pericarditis and then after several months of tests, [something called] giant cell arteritis (which is inflammation of the arteries going through my temple to the brain). The tests showed major inflammation in my body, so I was put on very large doses of prednisone. That caused many more problems. We have been trying to lower the dose for about six months and it has been up and down. I have had lab tests every two weeks for the last fifteen months. Then, five weeks ago, I began my lifestyle change mainly because it was touted to be good for inflammation and I had gained lots of weight with the help of

the prednisone. After the first two weeks into your program, my inflammation tests were still high, but last week, both indicators showed that my levels were in the normal range. That is the first time in more than ten years. I can't tell you how happy that has made me and my family. I am a believer! I feel good. I don't miss either the gluten or the sugar. I can't thank you both enough for the guidance and information. It just proves that you can teach an old dog new tricks. Thank you!
—Molly

Autoimmune Disorders: From Type 1 Diabetes to Thyroid Issues

What is really cool about this diet is just how amazing people start to feel. Certain diets that are known for counting "points" can't claim this. Sure, people may lose weight and be happy about that, but ailments are not cured. Dieters that count "points" do not get off their thyroid medication, they are not cured of depression, they are not sleeping better, and they are not getting the results that a well-formulated keto-adapted diet would give them.

I use to *love* Fridays because for me, that meant eating whatever I wanted. I was 80% perfect low-carb and grain-free, but on the weekend, I "cheated." I wasn't terrible, but a French fry here, a glass of wine there ... I wasn't comfortable in my skin. One of the most common complaints I hear from clients is that when they slip and consume junk, they feel almost hungover the next day. I've been on a lot of diets in my day, and what I find interesting is that the hungover feeling doesn't happen on low-fat, "whole grain"-filled diets. Sure, you may feel depressed because the scale goes up after a bender of donuts, but you don't get the physical illness.

This is why the keto-adapted way of eating is so powerful! If you go all in, amazing results happen. Only once you go all in do you start to realize how low your energy was. I say "all in" because just like Dr. William Davis of *Wheat Belly* explains, you can't cut wheat 80 percent and expect 80 percent results. It doesn't work that way. It needs to be 100 percent. You can "diet" on the weekdays, then "cheat" on the weekends, if you like. But I no longer feel the need to cheat with the meals I'm eating!

Cutting the wheat and sugar isn't a diet for me. It is a lifestyle. I love food and I will always love food, but more so, I love the way I feel when I eat like this! That is why I spend so much time and money experimenting with new recipes for all of you. I want you to be able to do this 100 percent.

If you also decide to make this way of eating your lifestyle, you'll notice you no longer want to nap in the afternoon, the belly fat will disappear, your skin will look amazing, joint pain is no longer an issue, and you will no longer be hungry all day or be thinking about food. Sure, it takes time to plan and prepare meals, but we all make priorities with our time. When you feel and look amazing, you will never regret the time you put into it.

Craig has been gluten and sugar free for about three years now. What I never thought he would cut out is beer. He was a beer connoisseur — he even brewed his own beer. When he cut out beer, he started making his own wine. But knowledge is power and the more he learned, the more he didn't want to even have a glass of wine a week. After being gluten free and fructose free for many months, your body stops producing antibodies and you start to feel amazing; this is how Craig felt. But one day, we were having a celebration and he had a glass of wine. That was the only thing that he changed about his diet. Immediately he felt a "dumping" effect starting, and sure enough, fructose malabsorption. He never realized his immune response to fructose until he cut it out 100% for a very long period of time.

I really believe that people think they feel fine, but it isn't until you cut certain foods that are causing immune responses and antibodies to be high that you really start to feel amazing!

I refer to this diet as "well-formulated" because if you just attempt a low-carb diet and don't cut out inflammatory "low-carb" foods such as gluten (the protein found in wheat) or dairy, you are not likely going to notice much of a difference. Many low-carb cookbooks use ingredients that are low-carb, but often contain substances that cause an autoimmune response, which causes thyroid disorders, multiple sclerosis, alopecia, arthritis, Addison's disease, vertigo, autism, hemolytic anemia, Colitis, Crohn's disease, chronic fatigue syndrome, type 1 diabetes, Parkinson's, Sjogren's syndrome, and any other autoimmune disorder.

Celiac Disease: The "Gateway" Autoimmune Initiator

"Where's the closest bathroom?" was the first question that would come out of my mouth when we would step foot into a restaurant. From as early as I can remember, I have suffered from horrible stomach pains after eating meals. I always laughed off my "digestive issues" until one day my two-year-old daughter saw me holding my stomach in the fetal position on the couch after a "fun" night out for dinner. She worriedly asked my husband, "What's wrong with Mommy?" I knew at that point I had to get some answers and so I began the very long road to healing my gut. I was referred to a gastroenterologist who told me that although my gallbladder was functioning at a healthy rate, it should be removed. I was not keen on having an organ taken out of my body, so instead he told me to stay away from butter and oils. I did just that ... and lived on boring salads with low-fat dressing for years. Yes, my stomach pains did go away, but my diet was so boring! Then, slowly but surely, I started to get sick again. First it was pneumonia, then nearly once a month I would get almost flu-ish and end up in bed. My weight started to fluctuate, too, but the last straw was when I came down with shingles. I knew, at 28, that something bad was going on in my body. My doctor told me not to worry, and shingles were completely normal in a twenty-eight-year-old woman. It was just too much "stress" in my life ... but I wasn't stressed! Then one night (when I couldn't sleep due to the steroids they pumped in me to combat the shingles) I was researching my issues and came across celiac disease. My mind raced as every description matched mine. The next day I made a conscious decision to cut out wheat. I was ecstatic! I immediately felt a difference in my energy, moods, etc. After a month of eating gluten-free, I decided to contact my doctor and get a test to "confirm" my allergy. He reluctantly did the tests and cheerfully called me the next week to tell me I didn't have celiac ... but possibly a gluten "sensitivity." I was crushed! I thought I had found the answer to all my problems. But, as Maria points out, there is a large percentage of false negatives when tested for celiac.

Fast forward to today. I am ever so grateful to have met Maria! I try to adhere to a ketogenic diet, which means high-fat (butter and oils, gasp!), moderate protein and low-carb foods. I have never enjoyed such a wide array of foods in my entire life! Eating is now fun again. My stomach issues have completely disappeared, but what's more astonishing are the other changes: my clearer thinking, my muscle definition, my energy levels, my skin, my moods. The list goes on and on. I am a group fitness instructor and most days of the week I need to be in the gym all morning strength training and teaching high-intensity cardio. I usually don't get home until late afternoon and a ketogenic diet allows me to have the energy to do this! I sometimes even need to remind myself to eat!

And my Raynaud's syndrome completely disappeared! This photograph is evidence of what my husband used to refer to as my "corpse" fingers. For eight months out of the year, I would lose complete feeling in not only all of my fingers, but my toes and nose as well! My husband even bought me a very expensive pair of boots that I would clomp around in ... and that still didn't work. I would spend 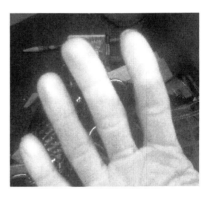 *hours just focusing on trying to get blood back into my fingers, to no avail. Out of the blue one day, after switching to a high-fat diet, I suddenly realized I have not lost any feeling since! It's crazy!*

One other "plus": I have been addicted to Diet Mountain Dew since college (over 10 years ago). I used to say, "If you want to kill me, lock me in a room without Diet Dew." I would drink six cans a day. I was so proud of myself when I cut down to four! After eating this way, I suddenly felt ill whenever I would try to slug a can. So I completely quit my pop addiction cold-turkey. The weird thing is, my body doesn't need the caffeine! The fats in my diet drive my energy sky-high. Now, if you would have told me I wouldn't drink pop five years ago, I would have died laughing!

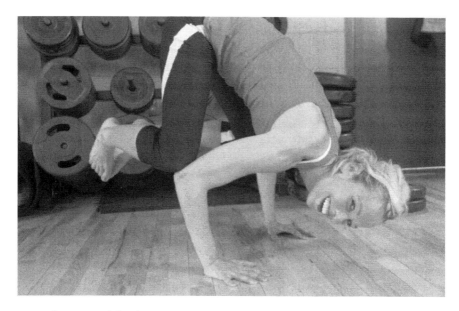

I am forever indebted to Maria for opening my horizons to the ketogenic diet and for freeing me from a life of boring salads!

—Kristen

Dr. Perlmutter, author of *Grain Brain*, discusses gluten and casein (the protein found in wheat and dairy) and their impact on autoimmune diseases. He also discusses how glucose (sugar) and carbohydrates play a powerfully toxic role in one's diet. Dr. Perlmutter also describes how a gluten sensitivity is involved in almost all chronic diseases because of how gluten affects your immune system. Unfortunately, the majority of people (including the medical community) still mistakenly believe that if you don't have celiac disease, gluten is fair game, and you can eat as much of it as you like.

True celiac disease, which is gluten sensitivity affecting your small intestine, affects around 1.8 percent of people in the United States. But a gluten sensitivity may actually affect as much as 30 to 40 percent of people, and some doctors, such as Dr. Alessio Fasano at Massachusetts General Hospital, believes that we all are affected by gluten to some degree.

I believe everyone should cut gluten because we all create something called zonulin in the intestine in response to gluten. When you ingest gluten, it makes your gut more penetrable, which then allows proteins to get into your bloodstream that would not be allowed in if the gut were healthy. This, in turn, causes your autoimmune system to go into overdrive and promotes inflammation and autoimmune disorders.

There are numerous differences between food allergies and full blown auto-immune disorders. The immune system's job is to free the body of foreign substances that might be damaging to it, such as viruses and bacteria. It also builds protection against these invaders if they try to attack again. This process is referred to "the immune response." The immune response can also react incorrectly to the body's own normal tissues. Basically, the immune system believes that a part of the body is a foreign substance. It attacks the body's tissues, a process called an autoimmune response. This occurs in autoimmune disorders such as Hashimoto's, Graves' disease, celiac, rheumatoid arthritis, multiple sclerosis, and lupus. Problems arise when the body overreacts so aggressively that it creates symptoms called an allergic reaction; the foreign element that triggers the allergic reaction is considered an allergen.

Celiac disease (CD) is an autoimmune disorder caused by the ingestion of gluten. In celiac disease, gluten stimulates the production of immunoglob-ulins that attack the villi lining the small intestine. Celiac disease is often confused for an allergic illness because like an allergy, it requires a foreign substance to generate it. Celiac disease is not a wheat allergy nor is it a gluten allergy. Many cases of CD are asymptomatic; the gut morphological changes may be minimal, so it cannot be recognized.[51] Let me clarify what I mean about the differences between celiac and a wheat allergy. Untreated celiac disease causes the activation of a type of white blood cell called the T lymphocyte (or T cell) along with other parts of the immune system, an activation which increases the risk of gastrointestinal lymphomas. A wheat allergy would not cause any of these problems.

Another difference between autoimmune conditions and allergies is that autoimmune disorders are never outgrown: they persist for life. Allergies can sometimes be outgrown.[52] If caught early enough, and action is taken by eliminating gluten 100% from your diet, you can eliminate the other autoimmune disorders that you may be suffering from due to celiac.[51]

Celiac disease is characterized by the presence of antibodies, which is why I always send my clients to get a "full panel thyroid test *with* antibodies," a test that is never typically run unless asked for or begged for. These antibodies are called antigliadin, anti-endomysium, and antireticulin.

The incidence of celiac in autoimmune disorders has been shown to be increasing up to thirty-fold in comparison to the general population, and in many cases it occurs silently with no symptoms. The identification of silent celiac is imperative: celiac has been found to be the gateway disorder to other autoimmune disorders such as autoimmune thyroid (Hashimoto's or Graves'), type I diabetes, and other endocrine ailments.

I often get asked why celiac disease happens in some people. There is some confusion about what really causes it. One theory is that celiac disease is triggered after an infection by a type of virus that biologically resembles gluten. After the infection, the body can no longer differentiate between the invading virus and gluten, which causes the body to react by releasing mucous into the intestinal tract upon gluten exposure and by causing damage to the intestines. This is considered "molecular mimicry." It's important to understand that, even if the bacteria or virus triggering the attack is removed, the autoimmunity never turns off. So the body continues to produce antibodies and attack healthy tissue even though the primary trigger is gone.

Molecular mimicry has been shown to start the snowball of the autoimmune responses. The theory is that molecular mimicry is actually the result of autoimmune disease, not a cause of the autoimmunity. That tells us that molecular mimicry is definitely a factor in the progression of preexisting conditions that trigger autoimmune disease, but that something else is responsible for triggering it in the first place.

With celiac disease, we know that gluten (a non-self antigen) finds its way inside the body and causes cross-reaction, but this evolution in thinking shows this to be only an effect of other preexisting conditions.[3] This is important to note because in order to heal, we need to discover what else is confusing the immune system.

It is disturbing to find that 60% of adults never completely heal from celiac disease despite following a gluten-free diet.[53] Another study found that only 8% of adult patients with celiac disease eating a gluten-free diet reached "normalization," where their intestines completely recovered.

However, there is new research that may help people with celiac for good! Researcher Alessio Fasano, M.D. has been on the leading edge of recent autoimmune and celiac disease exploration. In 2011, he published a paper titled "Leaky Gut and Autoimmune Diseases" which presented a new theory that suggests prevention and reversal of autoimmune disease is possible. He finds that there are two reasons for autoimmune responses:

1. An exposure to an environmental trigger
   - gluten = celiac disease
2. A genetic predisposition to autoimmunity
   - HLA DQ2/DQ8 genes = celiac disease
3. "Leaky gut," also called increased intestinal permeability

The reason why this is so helpful for healing is that by combining this knowledge, we can heal. We need to not only get rid of the trigger, but we also need to heal the leaky gut. That means we need to heal the gut tissue and restore intestinal permeability and the finger-like villi in the intestines in order to fully function again. This kind of gut permeability is also promoted by things like antibiotics and chlorinated water.

This new information tells us that if you have celiac disease, you also have leaky gut. Leaky gut causes other proteins found in foods to leak into your blood stream. This is detrimental because the blood doesn't recognize this foreign substance and attacks it, causing the autoimmune response to continue. In some cases, eliminating other common allergens, such as dairy and eggs (which are usually things I love on low-carb diets), needs to be done in case those are causing a response, too.

To heal the leaky gut, things like L-glutamine, good gut bacteria, and aloe vera help to speed the healing. This is also why I am on a keto-adapted diet. It is anti-inflammatory. If you are eating excess sugar and starch, you keep the gut in an inflammatory state, which causes an inability to heal. "Gluten-free" foods at the supermarket, such as rice pasta, was the worst thing to happen to people with celiac disease. Rice flour, the common substitute for wheat, has about 100 more calories and has 50 more grams of carbohydrates per cup than white flour. This is a recipe for inflammation of the gut.

Type 1 Diabetes

I am a type 2 [diabetic] and I found "my Maria" in my city; she put me on a sugar-free, gluten-free, dairy-free plan. I am no longer on insulin, plus I lost 50 pounds in five months.
—Crystal

Before we get into type 1 diabetes, I want to say a few things about type 2 diabetes. The single most important thing for type 2 diabetics is carbohydrate as well as protein restriction. This has been proven in any clinical trial you may study. In fact, most type 2 diabetics can be off of insulin within two to six weeks of being on a well-formulated keto-adapted diet. I've had many clients with type 2 diabetes who went from needing over 180 units of insulin per day to requiring absolutely no insulin within weeks. Not only do they lose weight, but they feel amazing, and their risk of heart disease drops immensely! Here is a diabetes testimony from a client:

I had another "Maria Moment" … this one was with diabetes. I have had my own success story with Maria's eating style, so I decided to introduce her recipes to my very picky, very diabetic father-in-law. I spend the summers at the lake with my in-laws and decided that this year I was going to cook out of Maria's cookbook exclusively. I made some of my favorite banana walnut muffins and almond waffles and asked my father-in-law if he would please try some. He is not fond of trying new foods, maybe due to being picky, but also because he has had terrible diabetes for over thirty years. My father-in-law has large blood sugar swings even with his insulin pump.

He tried the waffles and muffins and loved them. Keep in mind he had butter on both and sugar-free syrup on the waffle. As we stood in the kitchen discussing how many units of insulin he should calculate for the food he ate, we came to the conclusion that he should take 5 units. Normally for the food he had just consumed, he would have needed to take 8 but since Maria's food is different, we shot it on the lower side. My father-in-law left for about an hour then came back out of sorts. My mother-in-law said, "Tom, are you OK? Go check your blood." He went and checked his blood and it had taken a huge nose dive … he had a blood sugar level of 45! Now at this time only 2 units had gone into his body, not 5. He had to stop the rest of the insulin from entering his system. We couldn't believe it! Here he had taken almost four times less than he normally would have and his levels were too low.

OK, fast forward … About a week later, his blood sugar was too low, so my mother-in-law said, "Tom, why don't you have two almond waffles with butter and syrup to bring your blood sugars up a bit." He decided he would do this but they had to decide how much insulin he should take … what they decided was that he would take nothing! Now how crazy does that sound. In all the years I have known him, which is twenty-eight years, I have never seen him not adjust his levels when he eats something. So, Tom ate the waffles and I hung out to see what happened, and after about an hour and a half his levels were back in the normal range. Not only did he not have to take any insulin, but his levels were taking care of what needed to be done without huge swings and without adjusting for the food. It was so cool! Now, it's on to trying more of Maria's recipes and working with his levels. But after these results, my father-in-law is a believer in these recipes. Maria's way of eating does change lives … even lives that have known only diabetes for years. Thank you again, Maria, for your help … here is just another moment where you have made a positive effect on someone's life. You rock, girl!
—Cindy V (Northfield, MN)

I have worked with many clients with type 1 diabetes, and it is also the case that you can significantly reduce their insulin requirement when you reduce the amount of carbohydrates and protein they're consuming. Remember, too much protein turns into sugar via gluconeogenesis, so what's left? Fat, fat, fat! But type 1 diabetes is also caused by an immune response, so it is critical to also cut out the food causing the sensitivity or allergy that in turn causes this response. One of my clients is a physician in Europe and is now an extremely well-controlled type 1 diabetic after we changed her diet. She was able to reduce her need for insulin (both bolus and basal types) by almost 80%. Another client with type 1 diabetes came to me while needing 250 units of insulin a day, and within a month of eating a well-formulated keto-adapted diet, he was able to decrease his insulin to 20 units a day.

I get a lot of type 1 diabetics that comment or write to me saying that I need to remember to say type 2 diabetes when I write about carbohydrates and my success stories. I understand the differences between type 1 and type 2, but a well-formulated keto-adapted diet does help type 1 also! Type 1 diabetes develops when antibodies destroy the cells in the pancreas that produce and secrete insulin. The body normally produces these antibodies to defend itself from foreign invaders, but sometimes these helpful antibodies turn on the body's own cells. In the case of type 1 diabetes, the antibodies target the pancreatic cells. Most of the time, these antibodies can be identified through the examination of a blood sample. When antibodies are present in the blood, it means the blood is attacking a foreign substance. When food leaks from the intestines into the bloodstream (because of leaky gut), the blood reacts by attacking the protein found in foods, such as the gluten found in wheat or the casein found in dairy. In this case, we need to lower the autoimmune response as well as count carbohydrates and excess protein. This is why a high-fat, moderate-protein, low-carb and allergen-free diet works for autoimmune disorders. There have been several studies proving an association between type 1 diabetes and celiac disease[51], so when eliminating gluten, carbs, and excess protein, I have some awesome results.

If you are a type 1 diabetic and you start to eat a well-formulated keto-adapted diet, it is extremely important to work closely with your doctor. When clients tell me that their doctor told them, "Don't worry, eat whatever you want, just make sure you cover your glucose with insulin," it's like saying to a firefighter, "Don't worry, pour as much gasoline as you like on that fire, as long as you cover it with enough water." It is absolutely dangerous and irrational. In this case, I suggest finding a new doctor who will encourage you to eat a keto-adapted diet while watching your need for insulin.

The following is a testimonial from a client with diabetes and her experience in the hospital:

I was flying from Toronto to Mexico about eight years ago. When buying my ticket, they asked if I had any dietary restrictions. I said I would like to have the diabetic meal, naively thinking that I would get something a little better than the rest of the masses. When lunchtime came everyone was served a roast beef pita wrap from subway: it had beef, cheese, and lettuce. Guess what they served me? A hot dog bun with lettuce and tomato! I couldn't believe my eyes. I refused the meal and said, "Are you kidding me, there must be a mix up with the vegetarian meal." They assured me it was the diabetic meal. I insisted for a roast beef pita because I needed protein. They were so confused that I changed my mind. Of course I threw away the bread from the pita.

The lesson I learned was to never travel anywhere without being prepared by bringing my own food. Thank you for all that you do, I have tried many of your recipes and enjoy them all!

—*Cindy from Canada*

Colitis or Crohn's

When you do an Internet search for Colitis or Crohn's, you most likely will find the "White Diet" plan. In this plan, you are not supposed to eat whole grain bread, but white bread. No brown rice, only white rice. The

White Diet consists of the following: white rice, egg whites, the white meat of chicken, white bread, white beans, and non-fat milk.

Let me explain why this is not the way to go. Colitis is a disease that causes inflammation in the intestines and other areas of the body. The overactive immune system of the colitis patient, and the daily bouts of diarrhea, combined with the blood loss during an active flare up, all drain the body of major nutritional needs, such as iron and vitamin B-12. All of this is linked to gluten allergies. Gluten in the gut causes an autoimmune response, increasing inflammation, pain, malabsorption of vitamin b-12 and iron. The intestines look like a "shag carpet" (the villi should be long and wavy). As you consume gluten, vegetable oils, and genetically modified foods, your intestinal "carpet" gets cut. You digest foods with your "carpet." As your carpet gets shorter and shorter, you start to have absorption issues like gas, pain, diarrhea, and other serious issues. You need to heal the carpet with a well-formulated keto-adapted allergen-free diet.

People suffering from this disease are also extremely depleted in good gut bacteria because diarrhea causes you to lose the bifidobacteria and acidophilus in your intestines; the loss of these bacteria causes flare ups to happen more often, since we need good gut bacteria for proper digestion.

HEALTH TIP: You digest dairy at the end of the "carpet," so a gluten allergy and dairy sensitivity usually go hand in hand. But if you grow your "carpet" back, you usually can start to consume quality dairy (not skim milk) again after you heal. Healing time will depend on how damaged your intestines are strict you are with your diet and supplement regime.

If Crohn's disease and ulcerative colitis are caught before serious damage has been done, both conditions can be treated simply by eliminating sugar and vegetable oils and by restricting carbohydrates. Carbohydrates, sugar, and vegetable oils are extremely inflammatory and are terrible for our intestinal health.

The main things to avoid are gluten and long-chain triglycerides. Long-chain triglycerides impair the healing time in active Crohn's disease. These fatty acids are substrates for inflammatory eicosanoid production. Polyunsaturated oils, as in red meat, have long been wrongly blamed for IBS. A study published in December 2009 shows that linoleic acid harms the gut, but news reports and health websites mislead by blaming red meat, which contains the least linoleic acid. It's the polyunsaturated fats and oils, derived from seeds such as sunflower, safflower, soy, and corn, that are the major dietary sources of linoleic acid; they are the most harmful oils for those with intestinal problems because they increase inflammation.

When it is absorbed in the intestinal lining, linoleic acid is transformed to arachidonic acid, which is a component of the cell membranes in the bowel. Arachidonic acid can then be converted into various inflammatory chemicals. High levels of these chemicals have been found in the intestinal tissue of people suffering from intestinal disorders.

Long-chain triglycerides come from vegetable oils. This means anything that is prepackaged: salad dressings, roasted nuts, "baked" chips, popcorn, crackers, cereal … you name it! We have been wrongly pushed to replace healthy saturated fats like coconut oil with harmful fats such as canola.

On the other hand, the MCTs (medium-chain triglycerides) that I discussed in chapter 2 are broken down almost immediately by enzymes in the saliva and gastric juices, so that pancreatic fat-digesting enzymes are not even essential. Therefore, there is less strain on the pancreas and digestive system. This has important implications for patients who suffer from digestive and metabolic problems. Since it is easily absorbed in the digestive tract, it also helps other essential healing nutrients become absorbed as well. Ulcerative colitis often begins with a virus or a bacterial infection; the body's immune system malfunctions and stays active after the infection has cleared. Coconut has antimicrobial properties that affects intestinal health by killing troublesome microorganisms that may cause chronic inflammation. Coconut oil resembles breast milk more than any other food and breast milk is one of nature's perfect foods.

People with the highest intake of omega-3 fatty acid ,also known as docosahexaenoic acid, reduce the complications of crohn's and colitis by 77%. Omega-3 fatty acid is found in oily fish such as salmon and sardines.

STEPS TO HEAL:

1. Consume organic bone broth. It helps with mineral absorption.
2. Consume coconut oil. In my recipes, I always give coconut oil as an option. It works great for baking.
3. **No sugar**. This includes starch, too. White rice consists of glucose molecules that are hooked together in a long chain. The digestive track, as we know, breaks it down into sugar.
4. **No vegetable oils**. Found in any prepackaged food, including cereals ("organic" cereals, too), roasted nuts, "organic chips," boxed meals, frozen dinners, and granola bars.
5. Supplement with L-glutamine, aloe vera, and other healing supplements. Take large doses of bifidobacteria for intestinal health.
6. Eat the "healthified," keto-adapted way of no starch, no sugar, quality high fat, and moderate amounts of protein.

Thyroid Gluten and Carbohydrates

I was diagnosed with Graves' and thanks to you, I gave up processed food, gluten, and sugar. Within a year, I was off all medication. If I slip up, I feel my symptoms right away!

—*Lisa*

We all would like to blame the thyroid when it comes to weight gain. The thyroid isn't just responsible for weight gain or loss, but it also contributes to how well we sleep, it produces stomach acid, can cause high cholesterol, and helps with absorption of nutrients. Studies show that the thyroid isn't going to make us gain 100 pounds; it really is only responsible for 5 to 12 pounds of weight gain if it is malfunctioning. But I do think it can have a "snowball effect." The thyroid causes you to be lethargic, which causes you to not perform daily movement like you would (exercise and even biking with your kids for fun). Instead of focusing just on weight, there are some serious problems that can happen because of a thyroid issue.

There are a few main causes of thyroid issues:

1. It could be an iodine deficiency. This is a simple thing to test and fix. Get your iodine tested if TSH level is over 3.

2. Excess bad estrogen in the liver and fat cells is a leading cause thyroid cancer. Excess estrogen blocks production of T3. T4 needs to be converted to activated T3, an event that happens in the liver. T3 is what makes us feel good. A supplement called EstroFactors helps detox this bad estrogen out of the liver, which will in turn heal liver function and increase T3 production for thyroid patients.

3. Excess bromide (I suggest a blood test for this!). Excess bromides are endocrine disrupters that can be found in:

   • Strawberries (due to the massive amounts in the pesticides sprayed on them)

   • Citrus drinks like Mountain Dew, Fresca, and Gatorade

   • Medications such as inhalers, nasal spray, and others

   • Bread (it is a dough conditioner)

   • Plastics

   • Other places bromides are found in: hot tubs, fire retardants, and swimming pool cleaners

4. Autoimmune disorders, such as Hashimoto's (underactive thyroid) or Graves' (overactive thyroid). Thyroid nodules, whether cancerous or not, are often precursors to autoimmune thyroid disorders. If I were you, I would request a run of my thyroid antibodies (test TPO, thyroglobulin, and TSI, if you have hyperthyroid symptoms). This often happens after giving birth. During pregnancy, the immune system

starts to change and circulate to protect the fetus. Once the fetus is born, the mother develops antibodies against her thyroid. In this case, adding 200 mcg of selenium while pregnant is not only very safe for the mother and fetus, but it also lowers the autoimmune response after giving birth.

The following is a testimonial from a client who struggled with thyroid problems:

Several years ago, I felt like I was dying. I was plagued by numerous symptoms. For example, [I was] always cold, no sleep, racing and out-of-rhythm heart, depression, hair falling out, and always sick with something. My doctor took the usual tests and told me that my thyroid was normal and handed me a referral to a psychologist. I was so discouraged, but found an osteopath that ordered a ton of blood work. It turned out that I have Hashimoto's, an immune dysfunction where your thyroid hormones are destroyed by your own immune system. I was on several medications. Then, a naturopath I visited told me if I would get off of gluten, I could kiss the meds goodbye. I initially just got rid of wheat, but through research and the help of Maria Emmerich, I have gone totally grain free and sugar free. Currently, I don't need any medications, which is awesome because I am super sensitive to prescriptions; there is always a price to pay. Hope this helps someone out there!

—Janet

Did you know that in 90% of cases, hypothyroidism is an autoimmune disease? Did you know that autoimmune thyroid disease is linked to a gluten intolerance? Hashimoto's and Graves' disease are most likely caused by a gluten intolerance. What happens is that the molecular structure of gliadin (the protein in gluten) resembles the thyroid gland. If you don't have a healthy intestinal lining, you can create holes; enter leaky gut syndrome. To review, leaky gut happens because food leaks into the bloodstream, and since your blood doesn't know what the substances are, it puts your immune system into overdrive to kill the foreign substance (this is why I have my clients get a thyroid "antibody" test; it helps determine if there is a food allergy). So if you are eating skim milk and cereal for breakfast, you will most likely have a dairy and wheat allergy.

The antibodies produced to attack the gliadin in the blood also attack the thyroid. If you continue to eat gluten, your immune system will continue to attack your thyroid. Some clients mistakenly think they can eat small amounts of bread or gluten on the weekend or at a party, but nope! The immune response to gluten can last up to six months every time you consume it. This is not an 80–20 type of dispute: you must remove gluten 100% to stop this from occurring.

In order to stop the destruction of the thyroid, you have to be 100% gluten-free. Gluten, even "whole grains," contains phytates that damage our intestinal lining and inhibit nutrient absorption. Many people make the mistake of running to their doctor for an allergy blood test to find out if a food allergy is the root of their problems. The main issue with this is that blood tests are about 90 percent inaccurate. Crazy, but true. If I notice a food sensitivity with a client, success comes by an elimination diet along with nutrition therapy of enhancing vitamins, minerals, and amino acids. It is also helpful to consult a doctor, but don't wait for a blood test to tell you what will make you feel your best; start now, instead.

If anything, I recommend a stool test. One in three Americans are gluten intolerant. In some clients with autoimmune disease, their immune system is so worn out that they can no longer produce many antibodies. This is why everyone should kick the gluten regardless of antibody test results. Focusing on symptoms rather than specific numbers, which can change daily, is how I like to treat my clients.

> **HEALTH TIP:** The higher your thyroid numbers, the higher your cholesterol is. This is because your thyroid interferes how effectively your liver breaks down and excretes cholesterol in the bile. So high cholesterol is a suggestion to get your thyroid checked.

It is extremely important to know what is causing the thyroid issue before you begin any medication prescribed by your doctor. If it is an autoimmune disorder, then you should work with a person like myself who knows how to treat autoimmune disorders. If you decide to just jump into medication, and then start to eat correctly to control the autoimmune response, you most likely will be taking too high of a dose. Once you address and eliminate what is causing the autoimmune response, we can most likely lower the dose.

If you take too much thyroid hormone and your TSH falls below 1.5, this can cause bone loss and other issues. Inflammation is a main cause of bone loss. This is why you need to address the *why* of your problem first.

People often ask me what the best medication is to take. Well, that really depends. If your TSH level is high, but your T4 is normal, then the prescription medications Synthroid and Levothyroxine are just going to give you more T4; this will help a little because there is more to convert, but it will not solve the problem. The problem is converting T4 to T3. This conversion doesn't happen in the thyroid, it happens in the gut and the liver. Levothyroxine and Synthroid won't help much. The medication Armour Thyroid would be better because it has T4 and T3.

If you have a problem with low T4, some people do better on the synthetic medicine (Synthroid and Levothyroxine) because of the fillers in natural medication (such as Armour). A few years ago, everyone became upset because Armour "changed their formula," but they didn't change the amount of T3 or T4. They changed their binding agents — just by doing that, many people reacted terribly. Some of those binders are cornstarch and gluten! No wonder! Those are common food allergens that can cause autoimmune responses.

In the case of a thyroidectomy, it is like removing gum from the bottom of your shoe. There is still some thyroid present. The thyroid is in a vulnerable area. In the case of Hashimoto's (cancerous or non-cancerous nodules), there will still be antibody production against that small amount. You need to address the foods causing autoimmune responses. Not only that, but your estrogen levels are most likely too high and unopposed due to a lack of progesterone. Detoxing estrogen with the cleansing supplements I have listed at the end of this chapter will be essential in total healing.

T4 Conversion and Low-Carb Diets

Now, what is really interesting is that in a few cases, low-carb diets have been found to lower T3 production, but scientists aren't sure if this is because people are consuming too little calories or if it is in fact too little carbs. I find that in my clients, it is linked to excess estrogen. T4 is converted to T3 in the gut and liver, not the thyroid. When clients have low T3 production, it is essential to cleanse the liver to make sure it is functioning optimally by cutting all sources of fructose and adding in cleansers such as milk thistle and EstroFactors. Signs of low T3 are excessive hair loss, low moods, and lack of energy (even when eating a well-formulated keto-adapted diet with plenty of salt and potassium for many weeks).

> **HEALTH TIP:** Many fruits, veggies, and other crops in the US are sprayed with cryolite, which is a pesticide that contains a high amount of energy-zapping fluoride. Today, Americans consume four times the amount of fluoride than we did in 1940, which was when it was added to drinking water to prevent cavities. It is found in many commercial products like soup, soda, and many other foods like black tea. Even the Center for Disease Control (CDC) has expressed concern that over 200 million Americans are exposed to extreme levels of fluoride. All of this is wreaking havoc on our thyroid. I would seriously consider investing in a reverse osmosis water filter to get rid of all chlorine and fluoride in the water you drink.

This is why I suggest rotating calories and nutrients for everyone. Adding in an "over-feeding day" (a day where you add 250 to 300 more calories of high-fat, moderate-protein, low-carb food) once or twice a week helps stimulate T3 production. Clients often email me after an "over-feeding day," saying that they were nervous about stepping on the scale that morning, but to their surprise, they were down a pound or two!

In extreme cases, we need a non-ketogenic day a few times a week to increase glucose and insulin levels in order to help the conversion of T4 to T3. Remember, you can make glucose from excess protein through gluconeogenesis. This is why an over-feeding day with more grams of protein is my suggestion, rather than increasing glucose with excess carbohydrates. To read more on how to add in over-feeding days, check out chapter 9 on "Helpful Tips for Success."

Thyroid, Absorption, and Supplements

A healthy thyroid produces stomach acid. If you are deficient in hydrochloric acid, you can't absorb the nutrients for bone health and thyroid function. A helpful supplement to take would be HCL with pepsin (500 to 700 mg caps) before meals. You could be taking a "magic pill," but if you don't have enough hydrochloric acid, you won't benefit from the pill's "magic." So focusing on your digestion is step one.

In cases where you have either the autoimmune disorder Hashimoto's or Graves', it is important to optimize your glutathione status. I suggest optimizing your vitamin D level (and you should never take vitamin D without vitamin K for proper absorption of vitamins and minerals such as calcium). A healthy vitamin D level would be in between 50 and 80. Labs will report to you that 30 is in the "normal" range, but it disturbs me that in all labs they determine "normal" by the average level taken by all the people that get tested in the lab. Who goes to get tests done? Sick people. A vitamin D level of below 50 is too low.

To get back a healthy thyroid, you need therapeutic doses of L-tyrosine, zinc, and selenium to help convert T4 to the more potent T3. Your thyroid is a mineral hog. It eats them up. My top choices for hypothyroidism are the following:

1 L-TYROSINE. It is a non-essential amino acid that plays an important role in the production of neurotransmitters dopamine and norepinephrine. In addition, because L-tyrosine is necessary for the synthesis of thyroid

hormone and epinephrine (adrenaline), L-tyrosine supports healthy glandular function and stress response. Tyrosine is an amino acid found in red meat and other animal products. It can also be made by another amino acid, phenylalanine, but it needs iron for conversion. Clients with celiac are low in iron due to malabsorption and leaky gut. Many women lack iron because of heavy periods or uterine fibroids. In cases with clients who are low in iron, their bodies can't make tyrosine and they may end up with low thyroid function. People who have stress use more tyrosine to deal with stressors, which also leads to low thyroid. Low thyroid leads to low blood pressure, cold hands and feet, and restless leg syndrome. Take 1000 mg of L-tyrosine twice daily on an empty stomach (1000 mg right away in the morning with a *huge* glass of water, and don't eat for at least thirty minutes. Take another dose mid-morning on an empty stomach).

2   ZINC. Take 30–50 mg of zinc at breakfast (TIP: As you increase your zinc intake, it can cause nausea. That is why I like this liquid zinc, so you can slowly increase your intake. Start with 10 mg a day for a week, then double it the next week, until you are up to at least 30 mg). Zinc plays an essential role in thyroid hormone function. Things such as birth control deplete you of zinc, and without the presence of zinc, the thyroid gland cannot transform the inactive hormone T4 into the active hormone T3. Another important role of zinc is that the hypothalamus also requires it to make the hormone it needs to signal the pituitary gland to activate the thyroid. If you are low in zinc, you are likely to have an underactive thyroid gland. Zinc is essential for a healthy immune system, sense of smell, reproduction, growth, wound healing, and blood clotting. If you notice white spots on your fingernails, have "back-ne" (acne on your back), have PMS, can't taste or smell your food as well as you once did, and your wounds take a long time to heal, I would add in zinc.

3 GLA. Gamma-linolenic acid, or GLA. GLA is an activated fatty acid that supports thyroid health. Because of overconsumption of trans fats, most people are missing the enzyme to convert GLA fats from foods and therefore must supplement with an activated GLA such as evening primrose oil, which will keep skin soft and supple. We need those fats getting into the tissues. I prefer women to take 1,300 mg of evening primrose oil three times a day to help with hormone balance.

4 ASHWAGANDHA . Take 1 cap (450 mg) of ashwagandha at breakfast and 1 at lunch. This extract enhances thyroid function and produces a significant increase in T4 thyroid hormone. It also works with guggal extract to improve the conversion of T4 to the more active T3.

5 GUGGAL. Take 450 mg of guggal extract at breakfast and at lunch. It supports complete thyroid health and enhances the conversion of T4 hormone to the more potent T3. Guggal and ashwagandha should always be used together as they have synergistic effects on the thyroid gland. Both boost thyroid without influencing the release of the pituitary hormone TSH. Ninety percent of hypothyroidism is due to a problem with the thyroid gland itself and not the pituitary or an impaired conversion of T4 into T3 in tissues outside of the thyroid gland.

6 SELENIUM. Take 200 mcg of selenium at breakfast. Selenium is essential for the conversion of T4 to T3, which is the active form of thyroid hormone. You can eat two to three Brazil nuts a day or, to ensure the proper amount, I recommend to take a supplement.

7 GLUTATHIONE . Take 1 cap of glutathione at each meal. It is a super antioxidant for your thyroid health and immune system.

8   RESVERATROL . Take 500 mg of resveratrol combined with 1 capsule of curcumin (turmeric) three times a day with food. Taking them together creates a synergistic effect, making them potent tools for quenching the inflammation and damage associated with Hashimoto's flare-ups and chronic inflammation. Examples of other inflammatory disorders it improves include arthritis, brain fog, gut pain and inflammation, multiple food and chemical sensitivities, fibromyalgia, asthma, eczema and psoriasis, and other conditions related to inflammation or autoimmune disease.

9   KELP. Take 300-500 mcg of kelp. The thyroid hormone thyroxine is 64 percent iodine. This important trace mineral is often lacking in the gland, and when it is deficient, the thyroid swells because it is overworking to try to produce thyroxine. This causes low T4. I suggest eating kelp, a super sea vegetable that is high in iodine. The salt in processed food is not iodized in most cases.

NOTE: *Always check with your primary health care professional before adding in any supplements.*

Rheumatoid arthritis

I am the ripe old age of 44 and have had Rheumatoid Arthritis for a year and a half now. Finally, insurance approved my $1900 a month Enbrel [medication] and that has helped, but I feel loads better getting grains out of my diet for good.

—Beth

Most people consider celiac disease to be a condition that only affects your gastrointestinal tract, but one of the many symptoms of celiac includes joint pain. In some cases, joint pain symptoms appear before any digestive symptoms in people who haven't yet been diagnosed with celiac. Rheumatoid arthritis is an autoimmune form of arthritis that can strike at any age and is linked to celiac. This isn't surprising, since having one autoimmune disease, such as celiac disease, puts you at higher risk of being diagnosed with others.

Even if clients test negative for celiac, a gluten-free diet is still recommended. Inflammation is the stem of all diseases, and gluten and grains become sugar in your body, an event that causes inflammation. Cutting gluten and grains = cutting sugar = stops inflammation.

Fibromyalgia and Chronic Fatigue

My heart goes out to all the people suffering from fibromyalgia and chronic fatigue syndrome. This is a debilitating disease that some doctors often dismiss. I believe, however, that there are many causes to this, and I have had much success with my clients who follow my meal plans and supplement regimes. Fibromyalgia (FM) is a disorder characterized by soft tissue pain and fatigue, which is ironic because even though patients are extremely tired, the pain causes an inability to sleep.

Vasoactive neuropeptides play a huge role in FM and chronic fatigue. In a healthy body, these neuropeptides are eagerly catalyzed to small peptide fragments that activate hormones, neurotransmitters, and our immune system. These neuropeptides, along with their binding sites, are immunogenic and are known to be related to a wide variety of autoimmune diseases. They play an essential role in sustaining vascular flow in our organs, control memory, and attentiveness, and they also control our thermoregulation. They are powerful immune regulators with powerful anti-inflammatory activity, and have a significant role in the protection of the nervous system. When this neuropeptide is malfunctioning, pain and other detrimental issues start to snowball.[54]

Vasoactive neuropeptides are also co-transmitters for acetylcholine. Acetylcholine controls the brain's speed and mental processes, keeping memory sharp and physical movements quick and precise. Acetylcholine controls activity in the parietal lobe, the area of the brain responsible for processing sensory information, learning, memory, and awareness. Inadequate levels of this chemical can cause forgetfulness, Alzheimer's, multiple sclerosis, dementia, dry mouth, dry skin, reading or writing disorders, speech problems, slow movement, mood swings, difficulty prioritizing tasks, and an inability to relate to others. Most women are predisposed to an acetylcholine deficiency because these symptoms set in with perimenopause. Estrogen and testosterone stimulate the production of acetylcholine. As levels of those hormones decline, so does the production of this brain chemical. This prompts symptoms like memory lapses, dry skin, and weight gain. The cholesterol in yolks help produce hormone levels. The reason why cholesterol levels go up after menopause is because your body is trying to produce more estrogen (which your ovaries are no longer releasing).

Let's dive into why a well-formulated keto-adapted diet helps lower the debilitating side effects of fibromyalgia and chronic fatigue:

1   INFLAMMATION. One of the reasons why so many people are dealing with inflammation is because of a rapid rise in blood sugar, which causes biochemical changes in the cell. Choosing low-carbohydrate and high–healthy-fat foods is one of the best ways to decrease inflammation. When blood sugar rises, sugar attaches to collagen in a process called glycosylation, increasing inflammation (and increasing wrinkles). Athletes also mistakenly eat too many carbohydrates that hinder their healing and recovery time because they are constantly inflaming their joints.

2   SUGAR/GLUCOSE/FRUIT. Sugar decreases the function of our immune system, which in turn increases FM and chronic fatigue issues.

3   HORMONES AND LIVER FUNCTION. Some ways we get too much estrogen is through exposure to chemicals that mimic estrogen, such as many plastics (microwaving food in plastic dishes or using plastic wraps and containers), and through eating non-organic food. Beef and chicken are typically given potent estrogenic substances ("super estrogens") to make them grow faster. People develop estrogen dominance as

a result of a high-carb, low-fiber diet; consuming excess fructose; drinking alcohol; having a "tired-toxic liver" (see my chapter on this in *Secrets to a Healthy Metabolism*); or through environmental factors — all of which we have some power to control. The liver is a filter of sorts. It detoxifies our body, protecting us from the harmful effects of chemicals, elements in food, environmental toxins, and even natural products of our metabolism, including excess estrogen. Anything that impairs liver function or ties up the detoxifying function will result in excess estrogen levels. If your liver is tired and toxic, a special diet plan is in order. EstroFactors is a product by Metagenics that detoxes the liver from excess estrogen .

4   CANDIDA. An overgrowth of yeast can cause muscle and joint pain, difficulty in concentration, chronic fatigue, neurological disorders, insomnia, bowel dysfunction, and a weakened immune system. These symptoms are very similar to fibromyalgia (or "fibro"). If you have been on antibiotics, have low moods, and crave carbs and sugar, you could have an overgrowth of yeast. A low-carb, low-sugar diet along with the correct probiotics will help to kill the yeast. Not all probiotics are created equal. And in that case, you need to eliminate foods that can cause candida to grow, even mushrooms, which are typically allowed on a keto-adapted diet.

5   EXCITOTOXINS. Monosodium glutamate (MSG or Accent, the brand name), aspartame (NutraSweet or Equal), and hydrolyzed protein are excitotoxins that overstimulate our brain and should be eliminated by everyone. They are found in just about every boxed and packaged food out there. Excitotoxins excite the neurons in the brain, causing them to fire so rapidly that they die. Once these cells are dead, they can't be remade. What is really scary is that when we initially eliminate these food additives, symptoms initially get worse as the body detoxifies.

6   PHOSPHATES. Most fibrous foods such as seeds, wheat, and oats have phytic acid. Many people with chronic fatigue and fibro have a genetic defect that prevents the kidneys from excreting phosphates.

The phosphates build up in the bones and eventually in the muscles, ligaments, and tendons. The high phosphate level damages cells' ability to produce ATP (energy) and causes the muscles to spasm. Coconut fiber does not contain phytic acid, and it helps improve mineral status when you replace wheat flour with it in your baked goods.

7   FREE RADICALS. An abundance of oxidative damage to the cells can cause fibro and chronic fatigue. When you are keto-adapted, there is less oxidative damage. As noted before, a well-formulated keto-adapted diet doesn't damage our immune system and creates less free radical damage in our cells. Free radicals are highly reactive molecules produced in the mitochondria that damage protein tissues and membranes of the cells. Free radicals happen as we exercise. But ketones are a "clean-burning fuel." When ketones are the fuel source, ROS (oxygen free radicals) is drastically reduced. Intense exercise on a high-carb diet overwhelms the antioxidant defenses and cell membranes which explains why extreme athletes have impaired immune systems and decreased gut (intestinal) health. A well-designed ketogenic diet, not only fights off these aging antioxidants, it also reduces inflammation of the gut and immune systems are stronger than ever. Restoring the cells and eliminating free radicals is essential and eating a well-formulated keto-adapted diet will do this.

8   MINERAL DEFICIENCIES. Magnesium is a miracle mineral that about 70% of people are deficient in (mainly because it takes 54 mg of magnesium to process 1 gram of sugar or starch). Insulin stores magnesium, but if your insulin receptors are blunted and your cells grow resistant to insulin, you can't store magnesium so it passes out of your body through urination. Magnesium, as we know, relaxes muscles. If your magnesium level is too low, your muscles will constrict rather than relax, which will increase pain and decrease your energy level. To fix this problem, eat a low-carb diet and consume magnesium Glycinate.

9   FOOD ALLERGIES. Having a food allergy, such as gluten, inhibits your intestines' ability to absorb iron and B-12, and both are essential for energy production. When we inhale, we carry oxygen through the hemoglobin to the mitochondria of our cells that burn fat and create energy. If we are deficient in iron, we can't carry the oxygen to the mitochondria.

10 NIGHTSHADES. Another possible source of pain could be from nightshade plants. Vegetables such as potatoes, tomatoes, peppers, and eggplant (all in the nightshade family) contain a chemical alkaloid called solanine. Solanine can trigger pain in some people. If you are unsure, I suggest eliminating these foods for one month to see what happens.

11 OTHER POSSIBLE REASONS. Not getting into REM sleep, an imbalance of omega-3 to omega-6 ratio, a damaged immune system, or parasites (which damage the immune system).

Alopecia

Alopecia areata is a condition in which the immune system mistakenly attacks the hair follicles. This autoimmune disorder is close to my heart. One client really sticks out in my mind — Kiki was a middle-aged woman who came into my office. I saw her often in the weight lifting class that I take three times a week, but I never talked to her. It was impossible to ignore that she always wore a bandana on her head, but I never knew why. Apparently, she started losing her hair in her 20's, and by the time she came into my office, it was completely gone.

I love this story because Kiki was a professor, so I never saw her at the gym during the school year. After six months of my anti-inflammatory, keto-adapted, gluten-free diet, Kiki walked into the gym with a bandana on like usual, and ran up to me with a huge grin. She riped her bandana off and had a full head of hair. She said with delight, "I had my first hair cut in ten years!" As a woman, I can't imagine. I use to let those "bad hair days" upset me, but after meeting Kiki, it just seems silly now.

Studies find a high rate of celiac disease in patients with alopecia; I recommend that testing antibodies for celiac disease be performed in all of my clients with alopecia areata. Aside from causing autoimmune hair loss, gluten causes leaky lut, which causes damage to the intestinal villi. This damage further depletes the body of vitamins and minerals that are essential for hair growth. This is why I also prescribe L-glutamine, bifidobacteria, as well as many minerals to help heal the gut and increase proper absorption so hair can grow back faster. My top choices for vitamins and minerals are:

1. Amino acids such as L-glutamine, which helps heal the intestinal lining. I suggest 3 grams at least three times a day about thirty minutes before meals or on an empty stomach.

2. Iron. I always suggest a "ferritin" test to my clients to see if iron is getting into the cells where it is needed. A hemoglobin test will not show this. Low iron causes hair loss, inability to oxidize fat as efficiently, anxiety, and sleep issues. Do not take iron unless you know your levels.

3. Selenium is essential for the conversion of T4 to T3, which is the active form of thyroid hormone. Low T3 conversion can cause hair loss. I recommend 200 mcg daily.

4. B-vitamins. Biotin (B-8) is necessary for your body to be able to properly metabolize fats. It plays a major role in energy production. Symptoms of biotin deficiency are hair loss, nail brittleness, dermatitis (inflammation of the skin), muscle pain, depression, and fatigue. Healthy intestinal flora or bacteria is responsible for producing 40-50% of your daily biotin. Those with long-standing gluten sensitivity are more prone to biotin deficiency for this reason. I recommend 50 mcg twice daily.

5. Zinc. is responsible for several hundred chemical reactions in the body, one of which is the production of collagen protein. Collagen is the

backbone molecule for hair. Zinc also helps regulate thyroid hormone production. Low levels of zinc are linked to hypothyroidism, which causes hair loss as well. Zinc is also necessary for digestive enzyme production, which are essential for the absorption of vitamins and minerals. I often perform a zinc deficiency test in my office, and more than 80% of clients are deficient in zinc. **Note:** I always recommend a chelated liquid zinc because as you increase zinc, it can cause nausea; please slowly increase your zinc. Start with 15 mg a day for a week, then double it the next week, and increase again until you are at 50 mg/day.

6. Vitamin C. This vitamin is vital for the production of collagen fibers, which are essential for hair growth. It also contributes to superior blood circulation to the hair follicles. Low levels of vitamin C can cause hair loss, anemia, easy bruising, lowered immune function, and increased risk of infections. **Note:** Most forms of vitamin C produced in the U.S. are made from corn, which is a common allergen. Instead, use oregano oil. I suggest 2 to 3 drops four times daily, or one 100-150 mg capsule (instead of the drops) three to four times daily.

7. Omega-3 Fats. These are called "essential" fatty acids because your body can not make them, you must consume them. Omega-3 fats are a vital component of every cell membrane in your body. They are important for keeping the hair and scalp hydrated. These fats also decrease inflammation. Dietary sources include grass fed beef, sardines, cold-water fish (farm-raised fish not included), and walnuts. I suggest 1000 mg three times a day in the form of krill oil.

8. GLA. Gamma-linoleic acid (GLA) is essential for cell structure and improves the elasticity of the skin. GLA contains potent inhibitors of type 1 and 2 forms of 5-alpha reductase and is highly effective in decreasing the levels of dihydrotestosterone (DHT), which causes male pattern baldness, acne, and excessive female body hair (hirsutism). I suggest 1300 mg in the form of evening primrose oil three times a day for women.

Summary

If this is scaring you, it shouldn't — you are in charge! Clients who come to me with autoimmune thyroid disorder can often get off of medication. Various antibodies that indicate celiac disease, such as thyroid antibodies, will disappear after three to six months of a well-formulated, keto-adapted, and gluten-free diet. This is important information for autoimmune patients, who are typically told that there is nothing that can be done to reduce antibody levels or to improve the "autoimmune" aspect of their thyroid conditions. Do not ignore this message, because if left untreated, celiac can result in long-term damage to the body. For instance, because celiac disease damages the small intestine, people with celiac disease are at risk for malabsorption, nutritional deficiencies, iron-deficiency anemia, and osteoporosis. Untreated, celiac disease raises the risk of contracting certain stomach cancers by more than double. Clients with autoimmune thyroiditis may benefit from getting a stool test for celiac disease so they can eliminate symptoms and limit the risk of developing other autoimmune disorders.

You are in charge of your fate — you can start to feel amazing and lower the inflammation caused by these antibodies that are turning on your body's own cells. Cutting out food allergens and cutting out inflammatory sugar and starch is going to be essential to healing your autoimmune disease. It takes a lot of planning, but in the long run, your body will thank you!

Chapter 8

Happy Fats

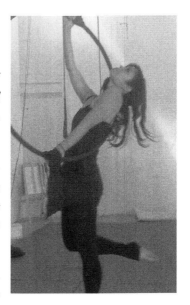

I started yo-yo dieting and exercising when I was 8 years old even though I was a slim child with no genetic tendency towards being even slightly overweight!

I had started baby ballet a few months prior and was so gifted a dancer that in just a month I was moved to the advanced ballet class with the older girls and was (apparently) even better than all of them.

My ballet teacher who was once a prima ballerina was so impressed by my ability that she pulled my mom aside and I had the ill luck to have overheard this conversation. She told my mom that if I continued to dance that I would someday be a prima ballerina assoluta. (I had to look up this definition when I got much older but at 8 years old I had no idea what kind of compliment I was being given). But THIS I remember...she said that for me to be a ballerina I would have to go on a strict diet because I was not a 'skinny' girl. That actually my (slim) frame was not ideal for ballerinas and it would hold me back. The ballet world would think I was too 'fat' and my body was not ideal.

There. My life was changed at that moment. I started a lifelong struggle with body image at that moment that I heard I was too fat. And even though I stopped dancing only 2 years later, the dieting and exercise continued. I would do 45 minutes of aerobics and toning in my room with my door closed and I was only 8 years old.

I never had an eating disorder but I was definitely obsessed with my weight. My eating was either feast or famine because I could never stick to a real diet. I had no concept for what was healthy and what was right. I went about 'dieting very blindly. And because I could never stick to an actual 'diet' i actually started gaining weight. All the feasting was catching up to me which made me try more starvation diets only to feast later on. Because i never lost weight and I would hide my binge eating, my mom never knew how obsessed I was with my weight and my body. No one knew. It was my own secret. To make a long story short, everyone in my family was thin except for me...which made me even more obsessed.

I have been on every diet I can think of and have been to countless nutritionists with little success. I was really at the end of the line and I always felt trapped in my body. I'm an emotional eater and have a major sweet tooth. Once I start I can't stop. I once went on a sugar binge that lasted almost a year. I felt like crap every single day!

Then one day, I had the good fortune to meet Maria who really understood me and my background! She showed me a lot of compassion and I knew she really cared about helping me.

She mapped out a great eating plan, but more importantly recommended supplements to curb my moods and emotions--which was at the crux of my emotional eating. Since then, I have bought every one of her cookbooks. I feel very educated about health and eating and can consciously make the right choices.

By the way, I have made almost every one of her desserts and ate it guilt free!! But I slowly stopped craving sweets altogether. When you don't deprive your body of something, it stops craving it.

Now, I am healthy at 5'6" and 117lbs and am no longer dieting or going crazy about my weight and body which had consumed the better part of my life. I can live and enjoy life the way I was meant to...something I haven't felt since baby ballet. Thank you Maria. You are a superstar and life changer....and forever my go-to gal. I love you!

—Romy

Fighting Depression with Fat

The purpose of this chapter is to show you that uncontrollable cravings for carbohydrates that keep you from achieving keto-adaptation are not your fault. Our brain chemistry plays a huge part in how successful you will be at adapting to the keto lifestyle. So if you are plagued by depression, anxiety, or cravings, this chapter is for you!

Before I started my job as a nutritionist, Craig (my husband) and I had some really tough curve balls thrown our way. I was a rock climbing guide and I loved my job, but with the bad economy came bad news. Craig lost his job which was our main source of income. Shortly after that happened, I went to have my yearly physical and I was a puddle. I cried at the drop of a hat, worried that we were going to lose our house and our dream of adopting children. My doctor immediately thought she would be a helpful "problem-solver" by offering me an antidepressant. She did not check my vitamin D levels (which ended up being low after I had them checked with a new doctor), nor did she check my liver health, which was also probably horrible with my high-carb diet at the time. Not to mention the fact that I was also training for a marathon, which added stress to my adrenal system.

My doctor also did not ask if I took fish oil or a probiotic. All of these should be a prerequisite for patients to test and incorporate before being offered these mind-altering, addictive drugs that have lots of side effects. We would save a whole heck of a lot of money on health insurance!

On top of that she did not ask what my diet was (this is the same doctor that didn't ask about my diet when I had severe IBS — needless to say, after this visit, I changed doctors). In biology class, we are taught that our blood is manufactured and begins in the bone marrow. In Chinese medicine, we are taught that our blood begins on the end of our fork. Yep, we really are what we eat.

One of the most common and serious ailments I see in my office is depression and anxiety. Our brain and cells are over 60% fat. With the trends and tips that health magazines and commercials push on us, it is no wonder depression is sucking us all down! Before my passion for nutrition came along, I had a passion for donuts. I was an athlete and thought I could get away with eating what I wanted, as long as I worked out. Not true! Even though I ate enough calories, I was starving myself ... specifically, I was starving my brain. Even though my stomach was filled with "substance," my brain kept telling me to eat; our bodies are smart, they make us crave certain nutrients we need. In my low-fat past, I always felt guilty about enjoying fatty foods. But the human body is hard-wired to crave cholesterol and fat because our body is made up of this crucial macronutrient, so don't feel guilty! You crave cholesterol and fat because they're critical to your health. When you eat real cholesterol and fat, your body regulates insulin levels and triggers enzymes that convert food into energy. Cholesterol from food controls your body's internal cholesterol production and protects your liver. Your liver governs not only how effectively your body burns fat, but it also governs your mood.

Signs of a toxic liver include weight gain, depression, cellulite, abdominal bloating, indigestion, fatigue, mood swings, high blood pressure, elevated cholesterol, and skin rashes. Many people struggle with weight gain and a sluggish metabolism most of their lives, and go through lots of yo-yo dieting unsuccessfully. You might be asking, "Why doesn't anything work?" You may have been tackling the symptom when you should be addressing the cause; weight gain is often due to poor liver function. The liver performs more than four hundred different jobs, and is the body's most important metabolism-enhancing organ. It acts as a filter to clear the body of toxins, metabolize protein, control hormonal balance, and enhance our immune system.

"Thank you, thank you! With your help, I am off the anti-depressant that I had been taking off and on for almost 20 years. Wow, I can't believe it! I had been convinced that it was something I was going to have to take for the rest of my life. I feel great; I still get a little emotional the week before my period, but it is manageable. In addition to that, I am off the Armour Thyroid. I will have my levels checked again in two months, but the last time it was checked I was holding in the normal range.

Also, when I started working with you, I was on the verge of having my gallbladder out. I am happy to say, I still have my gallbladder with no significant issues. Anyway, thank you again, I know if I had not found you, I would not feel so amazing!

—Casie

HEALTH TIP: The liver is where T4 is converted to T3, which is the activated thyroid hormone. Excess estrogen blocks production of T3. T4 needs to be converted to activated T3, a process that happens in the liver. T3 is what makes us feel good. A supplement called EstroFactors helps detox this bad estrogen out of the liver, which in turn will heal liver function and increase T3.

Your liver is a "worker bee" that can even regenerate its own damaged cells, but your liver is not invincible. When it is abused and lacks essential nutrients, or when it is overwhelmed by toxins and excess estrogens, it no longer performs as it should. Fat may build up in the liver and just under the skin, hormone imbalances can develop, and toxins can increase and get into the bloodstream. The liver metabolizes not only fats, but also proteins and carbohydrates for fuel. It breaks down amino acids from proteins into various pieces to help build muscle; this process directly impacts your calorie burn. It also transports amino acids through the bloodstream for hormone balance, which is critical to avoid water retention, bloating, cravings, as well other undesired weight issues. There are many different amino acids that have a variety of important jobs. For example, L-tryptophan is an amino acid that comes from protein, which in turn helps build serotonin. Other amino acids also help move waste (like excess "bad" estrogen); detoxification and elimination of this waste occurs through the kidney. These amino acids also perform many other functions, like building muscles.

HEALTH TIP: Speed up liver cleansing with milk thistle and sweating! Sit in a sauna or practice hot yoga. Just make sure to hydrate and refuel your electrolytes afterwards.

The liver's most important function, and the one that puts it at greatest risk for damages, is to detoxify the numerous toxins that attack our bodies daily. A healthy liver detoxifies many damaging substances and eliminates them without polluting the bloodstream. When we cleanse the liver and eat the right foods, liver metabolism will improve and we will start burning fat.

As liver function improves, so does energy. With more energy, fitness improves, because we have the ability to exercise more and improve our muscle tone. If you notice that you are more edgy, easily stressed, have elevated cholesterol, skin irritations, depression, sleep difficulties, indigestion, kidney damage, brain fog, hypothyroidism, chronic fatigue, weight gain, poor memory, PMS, blood sugar imbalances, or allergies, your liver may be to blame. The liver also plays a role in migraines. If this vital organ is overloaded with toxic substances, it can cause inflammation that triggers migraine pain. If you have tried many ways to improve your health and energy level and nothing seemed to help, it is possible that your tired liver is triggering your difficulties. Restoring liver function is one of the most essential actions you could ever do for your health. When the liver gets congested, it will remain that way and get worse until it gets cleaned and revitalized.

The following is a testimonial from a client with many problems including depression:

When I began my journey, I was size 3X. I had terrible mood swings and depression. I was diagnosed with autoimmune diseases such as fibromyalgia, idiopathic thrombocytic pupurra (ITP), osteoarthritis and asthma. I had fatty liver disease, high blood pressure, eczema, rosacea, skin tags and migraines. I am now an extra large, and I have no depression or mood swings. Though there is no test to prove it, I feel I no longer have fibromyalgia. I no longer use inhalers for asthma and I feel as though that has disappeared, too. The damage from the osteoarthritis unfortunately cannot be reversed. My low blood platelets from the ITP used to average a count of 30,000 and now sit between 70 and 80,000. My iron count averaged around 2 or 3 and I use to get infusions every 6 months. I now average a count of 10 and haven't had an infusion in over 18 months. A recent ultrasound shows my liver is now normal. My blood pressure is stable. Skin tags are gone, eczema flare ups are rare and my rosacea is better. Migraine headaches are a thing of my past. I haven't had a cold in over two years. I have removed 90% of prescription medications from my medicine cabinet. Nobody can convince me that this is a coincidence. I believe 100% there are health benefits to this way of eating.

—Terri

As we all know, being overweight can affect our mood, emotional well-being, and personal and family relationships. But what you don't know is that our brains and neurotransmitter supplies affect food intake, appetite regulation, and energy balance.

> For 90% of dieters, a deficiency in one of four essential brain chemicals can cause weight gain, fatigue, and stress. The solution to losing weight doesn't lie in deprivation diets; it lies in balancing our neurotransmitters. Specialized nutritionists, like myself, and advanced practitioners are focusing on how the brain affects our health.
>
> 1. Serotonin influences appetite
>
> 2. GABA curbs emotional eating
>
> 3. Acetylcholine regulates fat storage
>
> 4. Dopamine controls metabolism
>
> When these brain chemicals are balanced, our bodies are more able to lose those extra pounds.

Have you ever experienced any of the following: persistent feelings of sadness, irritability, tension, decreased interest or pleasure in usual hobbies, loss of energy, feeling tired despite lack of activity, a change in appetite with significant weight loss or weight gain, a change in sleeping patterns, decreased ability to make decisions or concentrate, feelings of worthlessness, hopelessness, or thoughts of suicide?

I see a lot of these issues with clients and they all can be red flags for depression. It is no wonder that one out of every six Americans will have depression sometime during their lifetime. Although depression is a real medical illness, many people still mistakenly believe it is a personal weakness. That "weakness" is a genuine problem, with roots in your body's brain chemistry. You can take charge of your life again by understanding and taking steps to balance your brain.

Depression has no single cause; often, it results from a combination of factors. Some of the causes may include nutrition, certain diseases or illnesses, family history of depression, difficult life events, certain medications, or excessive alcohol consumption. Whatever the cause, depression is not just a state of mind. It is related to physical changes in the chemicals of the brain. Everything in our bodies including our brain and its chemistry makes us who we are.

Too little or too much of any brain chemical alters our behavior, which can take away our happiness. The combination of these events creates a different personality, and in the end, changes our destiny.

So what causes neurotransmitter deficiencies? Here are some of the major reasons we can suffer from depressed neurotransmitter levels.

1. Dieting and Poor Food Choices: Not Enough Fat!

This is the most common cause of self-induced neurotransmitter deficiencies. Limiting fat intake or choosing popular "fad diets" that endorse their own prepackaged foods in order to lose weight restricts the amounts of basic building blocks (neurotransmitter precursors) needed to produce enough neurotransmitters. Studies from major universities, including Harvard, MIT, and Oxford, have documented that women on low-fat diets significantly deplete their serotonin within three weeks of starting the diet. This induced serotonin deficiency eventually leads to increased cravings, moodiness, and poor motivation. These all contribute to rebound weight gain, the most common, yet unfortunate, consequence of low-fat dieting.

Increasing neurotransmitter production during dieting is strongly encouraged to avoid yo-yo dieting. This is accomplished by taking dietary neurotransmitter precursor supplements during dieting.

2. Gluten, Leaky Gut and Neurotransmitters

Patients with depression or anxiety are told they have a chemical imbalance. I have found numerous clients who are suffering from mood disorders to be gluten sensitive. When they eliminate gluten from their life, they become a whole new person. But how could a food cause depression? Let's take a look.

Gluten is the protein found in wheat, rye, barley, and oats. Have you ever put flour and water together to make your own gooey paste? In Poland, they use this for wallpaper paste. I'm not putting that "gummy" paste in my body: it causes way too much inflammation.

Here is a testimony of a client dealing with food allergies and depression:

The very first time in my life I was asked if I liked myself, I couldn't answer. Yes, I knew I needed to seek help. This was the turning point in my life. I was 17 years old. I first tried traditional medicine: anti-depressants, anxiety medications, thyroid medication for my "hypothyroid" etc. but with little to no avail. I turned to nontraditional medicine. I was 20 years old. I was able to treat my illness through diet and nutrition, but I realize not all cases are that simple. I strongly believe that had I seen a psychologist before my lifestyle change, they would have diagnosed me as bi-polar. I was a mess. Sad, angry, paranoid, blaming others; something was always "wrong" or "a muck" but I never could put a finger on it. I would break down and cry throughout the day and I would always "come up" with a reason why I felt the way I did.

I first started by making dietary changes such as eating protein, less grains and less sugar. It helped some, but not enough. I then sought professional help.

At my appointment, I started to cry. I said that I don't know what's wrong with me, maybe it's just been a long day. Maybe it's all the testing and pocking and prodding. I remember feeling a dark cloud over me. I was told, "You're having an allergic reaction." I replied, "I am?" This thought gave me hope.

Once I started your diet, my cloud was lifted, my brain fog, my depression, my pain, my suffering. I was a "new person." I was my old self again! I was 21 years old.

After the lifestyle changes of diet and nutrition, my fibromyalgia, freezing cold all the time, and sadness went away. Things were finally "perfected" once I went 100% gluten free. Until I went 100% gluten free I kept developing new allergies. I was always bloated and constipated. I would still have occasional emotional unsteadiness.

With Maria's guidance of supplements and staying 100% compliant to her diet, my gut has finally healed, my emotional health completely stabilized, my acne gone, excess pounds gone, brain fog gone, and my tired / fatigue is gone. I am the healthy image I longed to be. It took time, persistence, patience, and self-discipline. It has been a journey that has paid off! I am now a wife and mother of three and have the positive energy they all need. I can truly be the sound and encouraging spiritual head of the home, focused on them and not on myself. I am now 29 years old.
—Lacy

After the digestive tract, the most commonly affected system to be irritated by gluten is the nervous system. It is thought that gluten causes depression in one of two ways. Gluten causes inflammation in the body. A gluten-sensitive individual's immune system responds to the protein gliadin. Unfortunately, that protein is similar in structure to other proteins present in the body, including those in the brain and nerve cells. A cross reactivity can occur where the immune system "confuses" all proteins in the body for the protein gliadin. This is called cellular mimicry, where the body attacks its own tissues, and inflammation results.

When inflammation happens in the brain and nervous system, a variety of symptoms can occur, including depression. Research shows us that patients with symptoms involving the nervous system suffer from digestive problems only 13% of the time. This is significant because mainstream medicine equates gluten sensitivity almost exclusively with digestive complaints. Please note that even though most doctors will dismiss a gluten allergy or sensitivity if you don't have any digestive issues, this is not true. You can have problems with gluten that show up in other parts of your body, not just the digestive track. Gluten can attack any organ: thyroid, gallbladder, nervous system, joints (arthritis), cellular membrane (multiple sclerosis), you name it.

> **HEALTH TIP:** As discussed in chapter 7, leaky gut is one piece of Celiac and auto immune disorders. Leaky gut is detrimental to our mental health because we need good gut bacteria to produce serotonin and other neurotransmitters. If the gut lining is damaged, you are unable to assimilate all the nutrients, amino acids, probiotics and prebiotics to build healthy brain chemistry.

In a study examining blood flow to the brain, patients with untreated celiac disease were compared to patients treated with a gluten-free diet for a year. The findings were amazing. In the untreated group, 73% of the patients had abnormalities in blood circulation of the brain, while only 7% of patients in the treated group showed any abnormalities. The patients with the circulation problems were frequently suffering from anxiety and depression as well.

In addition to finding circulation problems, other research looks at the association between gluten sensitivity and its interference with protein absorption. Specifically, the amino acid tryptophan, is essential for brain health. Tryptophan is a protein in the brain responsible for the feelings of well-being and relaxation. A deficiency in this protein can be correlated to feelings of depression and anxiety. Ninety percent of serotonin production occurs in the digestive tract. So, it makes sense that food might have an effect, either positive or negative, on serotonin production.

Our society is too willing to accept a "chemical imbalance" as an explanation for their symptoms. Instead of getting to the root cause of the condition, we simply swallow a pill — a pill that, in the case of anti-depressants, has very dangerous and undesired side effects.

The frequency with which clients can taper off their anti-depressants is considered "unbelievable" to many mainstream doctors, yet it happens regularly. How is that possible? Well, it is important to look at the root cause of the depression, rather than just putting a "Band-Aid" over the problem. Instead, I find success with a gluten-free diet as the main path to recovery, along with a therapeutic dose of amino acids, such as 5-HTP or GABA as well as vitamin B and other key nutrients.

Food allergies can also affect our children's behavior. Encounters with allergens stimulate the release of serotonin and histamine from most cells in the body. This stimulation alters arousal, attention, activity, and vigilance. As a result, a highly allergic child can be either quite sluggish or quite hyperactive, depending upon the system of the allergic reaction. Eliminating all allergens from the diet will eliminate hyperactivity or lethargy and inattention.

The increase in celiac disease might be because there is more gluten being consumed: "gluten enteropathy" is another term for this illness. Gluten is useful in cooking because it promotes a resistant, chewy feel to a lot of foods, including baked goods. But, as we increase our consumption of "convenient" foods (such as pizza, granola bars, and cereal) we increase the amount of gluten-containing grains on a daily basis.

When I tell clients to eat "gluten free" they often grab all the "gluten free" prepackaged foods on the shelf, but that most likely will cause more mood issues and weight gain and will slow the healing process in your gut. Rice flour, the common flour substitute in gluten-free products, is higher in calories, higher in carbohydrates, and lower in nutrients than regular flour. It can cause more inflammation in our body. So my recommendation is to make your own healthier options by using almond flour and coconut flour, which are very easy to digest. The healthy fats in nuts are actually nourishing to our brain. Nuts are also filled with iron. After first being diagnosed with a gluten allergy, you may feel tired; this is linked to an iron deficiency.

Gluten is the first allergy I look at when there are signs of a food allergy, but there are other common food allergies to look at as well. Dairy, soy, eggs, and fructose are all food allergies that can cause the same issues as gluten. If you suspect an allergy, you have two options: you can either eliminate certain foods for a two-month period to see what happens to your body and brain, or you can get a stool analysis to test for specific allergies. I find that most people stick to an allergen-free diet if they have the results sitting in front of them, verifying that there is definitely an allergy. Stool tests are not cheap, but are a lot more accurate than blood tests. Blood tests are 70 percent inaccurate. My suggestion is to invest in your well-being and get tested. If you discover that you are allergic or sensitive to gluten and you don't know where to begin, all the recipes in my books are gluten-free.

3. Hormone Imbalances

Hormones influence neurotransmitter release and activity. If hormones are deficient or are off balance, neurotransmitters do not function well. Premenstrual Syndrome (PMS) is a classic example of how low serotonin levels can temporarily shift each month. Mood, appetite, and sleep can be severely disrupted one to two weeks before the menstrual cycle. Another neurotransmitter, acetylcholine, decreases during menopause when dramatic changes in memory, mood, energy, sleep, weight, and sexual desire occur.

Saturated fat produces healthy hormones. Low-fat, low-cholesterol diets can be very unhealthy, especially for women. All our major hormones are made from cholesterol: estrogen, progesterone, cortisol, DHEA, and testosterone. If we don't eat enough, our bodies divert cholesterol from our endocrine system to use for brain function and repair. When that happens, it's almost impossible for our bodies to maintain hormonal balance. Hot flashes, here we come!

4. Prolonged Emotional or Physical Stress

The human body is programmed to handle sudden, acute, and short bouts of stress. On the other hand, prolonged, chronic stress takes a toll on the "fight or flight" stress hormones and neurotransmitters. Eventually, these become depleted and coping becomes more difficult. If you have ever heard of "adrenal fatigue," this is a terrible snowball effect for weight gain and emotional issues.

HEALTH TIP: Have you ever looked at the roasted almonds you grab for a "healthy" snack from the vending machine? I bet you would find MSG in the ingredients. MSG, an excitotoxin, causes damage to the neurons in your brain and has links to Parkinson's disease, Alzheimer's, Huntington's disease, and many others. Children are very susceptible to this type of effect on their sensitive and growing brains. Excitotoxins essentially overexcite the neurons in the brain; the neurons become exhausted and die.

Neurotoxins are also a main cause of seizures, though the damage may not be seen until many years later. When this happens, our neurotransmitters responsible for focus, mood, and memory have a hard time finding and recognizing their receptors due to the inflammation of the membranes in the brain cells caused by the consumption of MSG. Consuming MSG triples the amount of insulin the pancreas creates.

Brain levels of the neurotransmitter dopamine (important for mood and focus) are lowered by 95% when you ingest excitotoxins. But what is even more disturbing is that when you switch to being 100% free of processed food, your brain remains unable to produce normal amounts of dopamine in the hippocampus (the part of the brain most responsible for consolidating memory). This is one reason for the high rates of ADHD and depression.

6. Abnormal Sleep

Many neurotransmitters responsible for proper sleep, especially serotonin, are produced during REM sleep (around 3 to 4 hours after you have fallen asleep). Serotonin converts to melatonin, the sleep hormone. When serotonin levels are low, melatonin levels will also be low. When this happens, disrupted sleep occurs and less neurotransmitters are produced, causing a vicious cycle.

7. Medications

Long-term use of acne medications, diet pills, stimulants, pain pills, narcotics, and recreational drugs can deplete neurotransmitter stores and damage our liver. The use of ma huang (also called ephedra) and prescription diet pills use up large amounts of dopamine and serotonin. This can result in "rebound" appetite control problems, sluggish metabolism, low energy, and an unsteady mood.

8. Neurotoxins

Heavy metal toxicity, cleaning agents, hair chemicals, pesticides, fertilizers, industrial solvents, and recreational drugs cause damage to neurons and decrease neurotransmitter production. Excess caffeine, nicotine, and alcohol can also be neurotoxic. The street drug, Ecstasy, has highly detrimental neurotoxic effects. It can completely drain serotonin and permanently damage neurons, making recovery impossible.

9. Genetic Predisposition

Some people are born with a limited ability to make adequate amounts of neurotransmitters. They display symptoms of a deficiency as children and often have relatives who suffered from noteworthy appetites and mental illnesses. As they get older, affected individuals experience even more intense symptoms and debilitation.

10. Candida or Yeast Overgrowth

An overgrowth of yeast causes extreme sugar cravings and low good gut bacteria. Our moods come from our gut. Killing the yeast is essential to healing our brain chemistry and increasing moods.

Summary

If you are dealing with severe mood disorders, depression or extreme cravings, I highly recommend reading my book *Secrets to Controlling your Weight Cravings and Moods.*

Chapter 9

Helpful Tips for Success

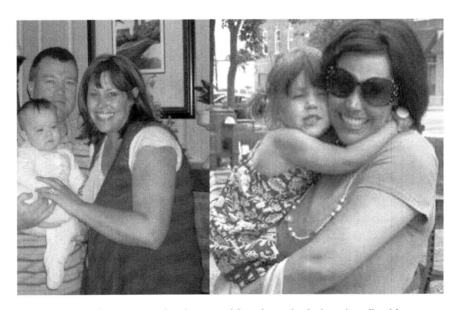

A year and a half ago I met with a doctor and found out I had a huge list of health issues . . . adrenal fatigue, digestive problems, severe candida, horrible migraines . . . and several other problems as well. To top off the list, I found out that I was also expecting my fourth baby (my oldest was only three at the time); my body was sick, depleted, and tired. Then I found you!

I purchased your health assessment and consultation. I followed your guidelines carefully. I saw amazing changes! (I am still working on healing my health after thirty years of damage!)

I very rarely get headaches. I don't crave sugar. I have lost all of the weight I gained with my babies! I feel great (most of the time! Four very small kids does wear you out!)

Thank you for your help! You changed my life!

With love,

—JG

E veryone is totally different when it comes to weight loss. Not one body is the same. I know there is a lot of information covered in this book, so I wanted to make a checklist of things for you to help you be as successful as possible in your keto-adapted journey.

1 GET YOUR LIVER AS HEALTHY AS POSSIBLE! The liver performs more than four hundred different jobs and is the body's most important metabolism-enhancing organ; it acts as a filter to clear the body of toxins, metabolize protein, control hormonal balance, and enhance our immune system.

Your liver is a "worker bee" that can even regenerate its own damaged cells! But our liver is not invincible. When it is abused and lacks essential nutrients, or when it is overwhelmed by toxins, it no longer performs as it should. Fat may build up in the liver and just under the skin, hormone imbalances can develop, and toxins increase and get into the bloodstream. The liver metabolizes not only fats, but also proteins and carbohydrates for fuel. It breaks down amino acids from proteins into various pieces to help build muscle, which directly impacts your calorie burn. The liver also transports amino acids through the bloodstream for hormone balance, a critical task that helps your body avoid water retention, bloating, cravings, as well other undesired weight issues.

Amino acids also help move waste, such as damaged cholesterol, used estrogen, and insulin, to the liver for detoxification and elimination through the kidney. The liver's most important function, and the one that puts it at the greatest risk for damages, is to detoxify the numerous toxins that attack our bodies daily. Working together with the lungs, kidneys, skin, and intestines, a healthy liver detoxifies many damaging substances and eliminates them without polluting the bloodstream. When we cleanse the liver and eat the right foods, liver metabolism will improve and we start burning fat.

As liver function improves, so does energy. With more energy, fitness improves because we have the ability to exercise more and to improve our muscle tone. If you notice that you are more edgy, easily stressed, have elevated cholesterol, skin irritations, depression, sleep difficulties, indigestion, kidney damage, brain fog, hypothyroidism, chronic fatigue, weight gain, poor memory, PMS, blood sugar imbalances, or allergies, your liver may be to blame.

The liver also plays a role in migraines. If this vital organ is overloaded with toxic substances, it can cause inflammation that triggers migraine pain. If you have tried many ways to improve your health and energy level and nothing seemed to help, it is possible that your tired liver is triggering your difficulties. Restoring liver function is one of the most essential actions you could ever do for your health. When the liver gets congested, it will remain that way and get worse until it is cleaned and revitalized. Speed up liver cleansing with milk thistle and sweating! Sit in a sauna or practice hot yoga. Just make sure to hydrate and refuel your electrolytes afterwards!

The following demonstrates the effects of the liver on our bodies:

1. The liver is where T4 is converted to T3 (the activated thyroid hormone).

   • Excess estrogen blocks production of T3. T4 needs to be converted to activated T3, a process that happens in the liver. T3 is what makes us feel good. A supplement called EstroFactors helps detox this bad estrogen out of the liver, which in turn will heal liver function and increase T3.

2. The liver breaks down fat if it is not tired and toxic.

3. This important organ not only helps you lose weight, but also controls your moods.

4. Remember this quotation from Jimmy Moore: "One way to remember that eating carbohydrates leads to an increase in blood and liver fat is to compare it to the French delicacy foie gras, a "fatty liver," created by force-feeding carbohydrate (corn or, in Roman times, figs) to a goose. The same thing happens in humans."

2 CUT OUT ALL DAIRY, EVEN "LOW-CARB," HIGH-FAT DAIRY. Skip the butter, cream, whey protein, cheese, yogurt, cream cheese and whey. I find that helps so many clients get to their goal weight. When you have

a damaged and inflamed gut, there is a phenomenon called "atrophy of the villi." that occurs You digest dairy at the end of the villi. So once you heal the intestinal wall with this anti-inflammatory, keto-adapted diet, you can incorporate those foods again (in smaller doses at first). I usually have people take L-glutamine and other things to heal the intestinal wall faster. This means no whey protein either. Jay Robb (my favorite brand of protein powder)makes a tasty egg white protein.

If this seems too daunting, cut dairy out for two weeks and then do an experiment: Weigh yourself the day before adding in some dairy and then weigh yourself at the same time the day after. Try to stick to lactose-free dairy with this experiment to make sure the weight isn't influenced by sugar (I would test with cheese). If the number on the scale goes up, don't panic; it's not actual fat gain … it's water retention. If water retention happens, then I suggest skipping all dairy for two months and adding in 3 grams of L-glutamine three times a day on an empty stomach to help heal the villi. Try the test again after you have stayed 100% dairy free for the two months.

3 OVER-FEEDING DAYS. When you add in an "over-feeding" day, I'm not giving you permission to have a "cheat" day of Pizza Hut and Dairy Queen. Not that you would do that anyway! But it is a "healthified" high-calorie day, ranging from 300 to 500 extra calories, mainly in the form of protein, so it stimulates gluconeogenesis and increases glucose. This event stimulates the thyroid. When you constantly eat a certain amount every day, your thyroid may start to produce less T3, the activated thyroid hormone.

We do need some sort of energy deficit, but if we do that every day for years, our thyroid may downgrade. This is why the "over-feeding" day helps. I don't recommend making breakfast your "over-feeding" meal.

This is indisputably contrary to the articles you read in health magazines that assert breakfast is the most important meal of the day. The fact is that breakfast may be one of the least important meals because skipping it allows you to enter a more efficient fat burning phase. If you want to take this a step further, you can boost your fat loss by exercising in a fasted state.[55] But let's discuss that in a bit. When you overfeed, I recommend chewing your food so well that it is pretty much a liquid before you swallow. I jokingly tell clients to chew thirty-two times before you swallow. I say "jokingly" because I don't really want you to count, but that number of thirty-two sticks out, and if you really try it, it is a lot of chewing!

For this reason, I don't recommend over-feeding days be big family gatherings. A lot of my clients choose Sunday family dinners to be their over-feeding day because of the enormous amounts of food served. But I argue that you should focus on the conversation and enjoy their company. Many times we don't even remember the food or the taste of it in large group settings. People also tend to swallow their food too soon in order to talk and join the conversation.

> **HEALTH TIP:** I prefer green tea extract capsules with little to no caffeine while eating because liquids dilute your digestive enzymes.

I personally choose my over-feeding day when I have a slower day at the office so I can chew slowly and enjoy every bite! The slower it enters your body, the lower the insulin response will be. Things like taking 200 mg of magnesium glycinate, 500 mg of vitamin C, cinnamon (capsule or free form), and decaf green tea will also help lower the insulin response. Keep in mind that that combination may cause loose stool. My over-feeding day involves a huge piece of crustless cheesecake with my 3 p.m. meal. I am not dairy sensitive, so that is my go-to meal that I enjoy over-feeding on.

4 INTERMITTENT FASTING. Breakfast isn't the most important meal of the day … "breaking your fast" is!

I remember when I first heard about "intermittent fasting." I thought, no, no, no. This is not good for anyone who wants to maintain their muscle.

But after diving into what happens when you fast on a well-formulated keto-adapted diet, I realized that not only do you maintain your muscle, but there are other amazing benefits as well. As I started putting this into practice, I not only experienced the physical benefits, but the mental benefits were outstanding! I now work and write early in the morning in a fasted state for about three hours and my mind has never been clearer.

Intermittent fasting came into my life almost by accident. With the increased amount of fat I ate (while also moderating my protein), not only was I losing weight, but I was no longer "hangry." When you are eating the highest nutrient-dense foods like herbs, spices, organic egg yolks, and organic organ meat, your cells are satiated.

Fasting is not a diet. It is a pattern of eating. You can eat very poorly while practicing intermittent fasting, a decision that will cause you to not reap as many benefits than if you were to eat a well-formulated keto-adapted diet. Fasting really isn't as drastic as it sounds. When you sleep, you are starting to fast a little. During first 10 hours after eating, you are digesting and absorbing nutrients. It isn't until after not eating for 10 hours do you actually get into a fasted state. If you keep your window of eating open to only 8 hours of your day, then after 12 hours of not eating, you get into a fasted state where you can burn fat more efficiently.

I know this may sound impossible. What I find interesting is that with most dieting, the mental part is easy but the physical part is hard. What I mean by that is knowing you need to cut carbohydrates and gluten is easy, but the physical act of making those changes is the hard part. With fasting, it is the mental part that blocks many clients from even trying it. It sounds impossible, so they don't even try. I was there, too. I did not like the idea of fasting or at least I thought I didn't. I liked eating. But since I was a sugar burner, I always wanted to eat. Now that I'm keto-adapted, I save so much time by not being plagued by thoughts of food all day.

The reason behind intermittent fasting is based on the foundation that your body tends to burn glycogen from your liver, but there is only enough glycogen for six to eight hours. Once your glycogen stores are used up, what is left? Fat! Yahoo! That is what most people are trying to get rid of, right? So after eight hours, your body is forced to start metabolizing fat rather than glucose.

> **HEALTH TIP from Dr. Davis, author of** *Wheat Belly*: "There are different genotypes that process cholesterol differently. The ApoE genotype[s] have about 99% lower liver functions and therefore are very sensitive to carbohydrates. LDL particles persist in the bloodstream for several weeks. This sounds terrible, but in a state of deprivation (fasting) this served you well, it provided energy for them. They were the survivors in our Paleo days, who could last longer when no food was available. There is also a genotype called ApoE [that] are incredibly adaptable to fasting and in our world of constant food availability, suffer great health consequences. Fasting is highly recommended for these genotypes."

When I read about how you need to eat every two to three hours in order to fuel your metabolism and muscles, I find it so ridiculous. Sure, if you are a sugar burner, you will need to eat that often, not only because you are "hangry," but because eating a high-carbohydrate diet burns up amino acids so you need insulin to increase muscle. But if you eat a well-formulated keto-adapted diet, it spares protein from being oxidized and therefore preserves muscle. Branched-chain amino acids (BCAA) are considered essential because your body can't make them, so you need to consume them for proper muscle building and repair (as well as for replenishing red blood cells). What I find so interesting is that BCAA oxidation rates usually rise with exercise, which means you need more if you are an athlete. However, in keto-adapted athletes, ketones are burned in place of BCAA. Critics of low-carb diets claim that you need insulin to grow muscles; however, with a well-formulated keto-adapted diet, there is less protein oxidation and double the amount of fat oxidation, which leaves your muscles in place while all you burn is fat! Athletes trying to gain weight can benefit from intermittent fasting, but it takes a lot of commitment to eating enough high quality food. You can eat during the whole window of eating if you are trying to gain weight.

Intermittent fasting is when you stop eating for fourteen to eighteen hours. Craig and I practice this daily, and in most cases, our fasting is closer to twenty hours; for some, however, this is too extreme or doesn't fit their work schedule. So trying to fit this in a few days a week is a great goal to strive for.

There are a lot of ways to add fasting into your life. For one, I suggest clients skip dinner once or twice a week. Maybe it is a day you know you will get home late and will be eating too close to bed. I like this because it stimulates the human growth hormone to be at a high level when you fall asleep. Some clients are so fat-adapted that they do this every day, where they stop eating at 3 p.m. This takes some adjustment. It is easy when you are a fat burner, but if you are a sugar burner and you continue to have a "treat" of sugar or carbs every once in a while, this is a hard thing to practice. Clients who are fat burners have emailed me to say that they no longer wake up hungry (or should I say "hangry").

FASTING TIP: If you are struggling to incorporate intermittent fasting at first and the hunger pains are too much, try taking 3 grams of L-glutamine with a large glass of water (or hot chamomile tea if it is an evening fast) and go to bed an hour earlier that night. The combination of the L-glutamine and sleep will aid your fasting efforts.

I like fasting in the morning, something that I practice daily. I wake up at 5 a.m. to work and I take my amino acids. Then I run on empty stomach from 8 a.m. to 9 a.m., and then eat breakfast. By doing this, I am well into a fasted fat-burning phase and I will only be burning fat on my run. I used to believe I needed to "fuel my run" with carbohydrates before I ran, but I never lost weight, even though I was running half as long as I do now.

Intermittent fasting goes beyond what Americans live like today. When I ride my bike with my boys, I pass other families and see kids munching on Cheerios and granola bars, and they aren't even the ones pedaling! I don't want to come off as judgmental because I was doing the same thing to myself. I was a sugar burner who would have to pack snacks if I left the house for longer than two hours. But it is so freeing to not have to stop and eat every few hours in order to focus. If this sounds crazy to you, think about our ancestors: they didn't have access to food every few hours, nor did they stop working to heat food to eat. Man, the microwave has made it easy for modern man, hasn't it?

Eating an early dinner and closing the kitchen is a great way to increase the human growth hormone (the fat-burning hormone) while you sleep. Our hormones are what ultimately determine weight loss or gain. They go up and down throughout the day like waves of the ocean. Insulin and human growth hormone are antagonists, and since insulin is the stronger and more powerful hormone, it always wins. So if you eat carbohydrates, insulin rises and therefore shunts the rise of human growth hormone. The largest natural surge of human growth hormone is 30 to 70 minutes after you fall asleep, but if you just ate a bowl of ice cream or toast with peanut butter and honey (which was what I always did as a kid), you stop that precious fat-burning hormone from helping you burn fat. By the time you wake up in the morning, you still have glycogen in your liver. You haven't burned any fat.

This is also why I'm thankful that I'm a morning person and always have been. I see clients who are "night owls" suffer from this problem the most. When we stay up too late, hunger can get to you, and your mind overwhelmingly thinks of food (and not typically of the things that would fall into the Pure Protein and Fat category… it is usually Doritos or ice cream). This is why you shouldn't keep this stuff in the house for anyone! Your kids, spouse, or house mates don't need that junk either.

Willpower is a muscle! If you are having a hard time with cravings, don't blame yourself. Willpower is a muscle in the brain that can get overworked. You *need* to limit temptations. You have only a finite amount of willpower as you go through the day, so you should be careful to conserve it and try to save it for emergencies. Work and family obligations may require all of your willpower, and you end up giving in to food temptations. I notice that if I stay up too late to work, my mind starts to wander to food; the thoughts become overwhelming. I know that if I had a pantry filled with junk, it would be too tempting. But since I live way out in the country and I'm not going to turn on the oven to bake, I take L-glutamine to help calm me and the cravings down and go to bed. I suggest you do the same.

Here are some more tips to help you stay the course:

1. Clean out your pantry. Other people in your house don't need that stuff either.

2. Don't put those temptations near you. Just putting food where you can see it next to you depletes your willpower.

3. Cravings, frustrations, desire — all become overwhelming. Make "healthified" brownies and "healthified" ice cream. I keep that in my freezer at all times! Especially in the summer, I feel the desire to eat the sugar- and wheat-filled treats that are going to set me off course … it is a downhill spiral!

4. In the short term, self-control is a limited resource. But over the long term, it can act more like a muscle. Practice, practice, practice = better willpower. It will get easier every day.

5. Supplements like bifidobacteria, L-glutamine, magnesium, zinc, and some others I have recommended all help with those nasty cravings and temptations!

Let's get back to fasting and why I love it so much.

WHY FAST:

BRAIN FUNCTION. A neuroscientist Mark Mattson found that intermittent fasting increases levels of a protein called brain-derived neurotrophic factor, or BDNF. This, in turn, stimulates new brain cells in the hippocampus, the region of the brain that is responsible for memory. (Shrinking of the hippocampus has been linked to dementia and Alzheimer's disease.)

INCREASES MOOD. The protein called BDNF that helps improve memory also suppresses anxiety and elevates mood. Mattson showed this to be true in a study of rats. He injected BDNF into their brains, and it had the same effect as a regular antidepressant.

INCREASES THE EFFECTIVENESS OF INSULIN, THE HORMONE THAT AFFECTS OUR ABILITY TO PROCESS SUGAR AND BREAK DOWN FAT.

REDUCES BLOOD PRESSURE. As your insulin level increases, so does your blood pressure. Insulin stores magnesium, but if your insulin receptors are blunted and your cells grow resistant to insulin, you can't store magnesium; it ends up passing out of your body through urination. Magnesium in your cells relaxes muscles. If your magnesium level is too low, your blood vessels will constrict rather than relax, which will raise your blood pressure and decrease your energy level.

REDUCES TRIGLYCERIDES. Insulin upregulates LPL on fat tissue and inhibits activation on muscle cells. On the other hand, glucagon upregulates LPL on muscle and cardiac tissue, while inhibiting the activation of fat.

WEIGHT LOSS. You burn fat, rather than sugar, in a fasted state.

INHIBIT CANCER GROWTH. Fasting cleans out damaged mitochondria. It "turns on" certain genes that repair specific tissues that would not otherwise be repaired in times of surplus. Studies have shown that intermittent fasting can reduce the amount of spontaneous cancers in animal studies, which is due to a decrease in oxidative damage or an increase in immune response.

LONGER LIFE. Fasting allows certain cells to live longer (as repaired cells) during famine since it's energetically less expensive to repair a cell than to divide and create a new one. Fasting reduces the amount of IGF-1 your body produces, according to Valter Longo at the University of Southern California. Less IGF-1, an insulin-like growth hormone, has been shown to reduce your risk of many age-related diseases, like cancer. You need adequate levels of IGF-1 and other growth factors when you are young and growing, but high levels later in life appear to lead to accelerated aging and cancer.

So how do you put this into practice? Here are a couple ways.

THE MORNING FAST AND EXERCISE. The purpose is to not break the human growth hormone and glucagon-dominant state dubbed the "fasted state." This works best for people who do cardio in the morning or afternoon. This will keep the fat-burning hormone (human growth hormone) high. Whenever you eat, insulin rises, which pushes the level of human growth hormone down. Your body will derive energy from food sources (calories) or from body stores (glycogen, body fat, and muscle). If you want to burn sugar, go ahead and eat before your workout, *but* if you want to burn fat, skip eating beforehand. A morning fast should last about eight hours. Do not feel that you need to eat right after your workout. If you are not hungry, do not force food, especially not a protein shake if you are trying to lose weight. This stops the fasting benefits. I suggest taking branched-chain amino acids if desired. This builds muscle without any calories.

During the morning fast you are allowed:

- Organic decaf Americano, tea, or water

> **HEALTH TIP:** Check your tea box ingredients. I have found gluten and hydrogenated oils in some!

- Small amounts of MCTs or fatty acids (fish oil), but stay under 50 calories. Dietary fats have very minimal insulin secretion rates. If you are susceptible to anxiety or adrenal fatigue, I suggest a quality fish oil to balance your brain chemistry and for its anti-inflammatory effects.

- Amino acids, such as L-carnitine, are recommended for whenever you wake up. This will help shuttle triglycerides to the mitochondria, where we burn fat.

THE EVENING FAST. If you aren't exercising, I like this fast a little better because it keeps you from binging later in the day. Consume breakfast and lunch, then fast for the rest of the day until the next morning.

During the evening fast you are allowed:

• Small amounts of MCTs or fatty acids like fish oils.

• I suggest 3 grams of L-glutamine to help with cravings and hunger when first adapting to fasting and keto-adaptation.

• Water, chamomile tea with no additives, or water from a soda maker sweetened with stevia

COMBINATION. Intermittent fasting should last at least eight to ten hours when you are awake. One way to accomplish this is to have dinner no later than 3 p.m. Then, for example, you go to bed around 10 p.m. (taking proper amino acids) and wake up at 6 a.m. When you wake up, consume only calorie-free liquids, such as water, green tea, or decaf Americano; I also take my L-carnitine at this time. I then recommend exercising at this time: I like to run from 8 to 9 a.m. I also recommend taking BCAAs and L-glutamine to repair muscles after a hard workout. You might eat at this point around 9:30 or 10 a.m. This process is a total of over eighteen hours between meals, with you being awake for ten of those hours.

5 STOP LOSING MUSCLE. If you continue to eat a high-carb diet, you will continue to be a sugar burner. As you switch to be a ketone burner, aside from using fats for energy, you will also prevents muscle loss because the need for glucose is reduced. Muscle tissue breakdown occurs when there is a need for glucose that exceeds the stores of glycogen. Fasting will also accomplish this. The dominant hormones in a fasted state (human growth hormone, glucagon, and adrenaline) are responsible for catabolizing tissue and can aid in the breaking down of fats from the glycerol backbone; these hormones also use fats for oxidation for energy instead of sugar. Adding in potassium will help maintain muscles, too.

6 EAT FERMENTED VEGETABLES AS YOUR CARB SOURCE. I often get asked, "If you think rice is bad, how can Asians consume so much rice and noodles, yet remain so thin?" The answer is that kimchi, fermented cabbage, and other fermented foods often start their meals. Good gut bacteria helps us digest our food properly and can assist with numerous healing benefits. It not only can assist you in your weight loss journey, but it can also boost your immune system. Eighty percent of our immune health comes from our gut, which contains over one hundred trillion bacteria, meaning you have ten times more gut bacteria than the number of cells in your whole body. A healthy body should have 2 pounds of good gut bacteria in the large intestine, but the majority of people have none due to antibiotics, stress, diarrhea, colonoscopies, or cleanses that deplete the body of this essential bacteria.

It's no wonder why I see so much depression in my office. The intestines comprise what is considered to be our bodies' second nervous system. You have the same amount of neurotransmitters in your gut as you do in your brain. When you are depleted of healthy gut bacteria, you become depleted of serotonin (the "feel good" chemical), which causes you to be plagued with thoughts of sugar and carbohydrates. Low serotonin also causes low melatonin, which causes poor sleep. I see this resolvable problem not only in adults, but the majority of children that I work with, too. Cravings, depression, and sleepless nights are not your fault and do not have to be your fate!

Kimchi and other fermented vegetables have good gut bacteria called probiotics, which help populate and rebalance your gut flora. Studies prove that probiotics can help heal a wide variety of ailments, such as depression, cancer, gut health, allergies, and weight loss to name a few.

Yes, a lot of Asian dishes use rice or noodles, but the nutrition of the dishes must be applauded! The bowl of noodles is made of homemade beef marrow bone broth, tendons, and tripe. They also consume large amounts of organ meats, such as beef tongue and liver wrapped in lettuce with a side of rice.

So start your meals off with fermented pickles, real sauerkraut, kimchi, or if you are like me and want to ensure proper gut balance, take a quality probiotic that contains bifidobacteria. With this tip, I ensure you that the cravings will subside, your moods will be much more balanced, and your sleep will be much improved.

7 SLEEP! Eight to ten hours daily. If you find yourself not being able to fall asleep, I suggest taking a cortisol test in the morning and at night to determine if cortisol isn't falling like it should throughout the day. I also suggest getting a ferritin test to determine if iron isn't getting into the cells properly. Low iron causes you to be extremely lethargic throughout the day, even though you might feel so anxious you can't sleep.

If you have trouble falling asleep, take the following one hour before bed:

MAGNESIUM IS A NATURAL MUSCLE RELAXANT. Try 800 mg of magnesium glycinate one hour before bed to help you calm down. Do not buy magnesium oxide; it is not absorbed well and will cause diarrhea.

ONE CAPSULE OF BIFIDOBACTERIA (PROBIOTIC). Bifido increases serotonin, which in turn increases melatonin production.

TAKE 750 MG OF GABA. GABA supplements decrease anxiety and emotional eating, increase mood, and shut off "brain chatter" at night; it is nature's natural Valium. GABA (gamma-aminobutyric acid) is a non-essential amino acid found mainly in the human brain and eyes. It is considered an inhibitory neurotransmitter, which means it regulates brain and nerve cell activity by inhibiting the number of neurons firing in the brain. GABA is referred to as the "brain's natural calming agent." By inhibiting overstimulation of the brain, GABA promotes relaxation, ease nervous tension, and increase quality sleep.

TAKE 200 MG OF 5-HTP OR 1000 MG OF L-TRYPTOPHAN. The amino acids 5-hydroxytryptophan (5-HTP) and tryptophan increase serotonin, which in turn increases melatonin output. **Note:** Do not take if on an antidepressant.

MELATONIN PATCHES. Many people claim melatonin doesn't work for them, which is most likely due to an absorption issue or leaky gut. I suggest a melatonin patch. Start with 1 mg and increase as needed.

If you find yourself having a hard time staying asleep and you wake up at 3 a.m. wide awake, the cause is most likely low progesterone (unopposed estrogen) causing estrogen dominance. In this case, I suggest you add a pure progesterone cream to an area of thin skin on certain days of your cycle. I prefer the cream Pro-Gest by Emerita. Many women in my office claim an immediate sense of "calmness" when I apply this to their wrist.

8 CUT OUT ALCOHOL. Doing this is very important for sleep, moods, and metabolism.

9 ELIMINATE ALL VEGETABLE OILS. Look at packaged foods: most use canola, cottonseed, soybean oil, or corn oil. Even "healthy" mayonnaise, salad dressings, and roasted nuts are most likely made with vegetable oils. Vegetable oils are very inflammatory.

10 DETOX BAD ESTROGEN. Do not microwave in plastic or drink from plastic water bottles. Eliminate non-organic foods laced with synthetic estrogen. Add in supplements to heal faster.

11 GO "NUMBER TWO" EVERY DAY! If you don't, estrogens get reabsorbed and locked into fat cells.

12 BENEFIT FROM THE "AFTERBURN" EFFECT. Wait a little after a hard workout to eat. When you work out, you increase the human growth hormone, which is stimulating the ketones. Once you eat, your fast is broken. The afterburn effect can stimulate up to four hundred more calories if you wait to eat. I suggest supplementing with BCAAs and L-glutamine to help repair muscles faster, then eat one hour after a hard workout.

13 NO SNACKING. If you are constantly fueling your body and increasing insulin, you cannot get into the fat burning mode. Do not eat every two hours.

14 DO NOT EAT TOO MUCH PROTEIN AT ONE TIME. You cannot store protein. Any excess protein will turn into sugar via gluconeogenesis. Split up protein throughout the day.

15 EAT SLOWLY. Eating slowly lowers the insulin response. It also helps register the hormone leptin that gives you the signal that you are full.

16 CHEW 32 TIMES BEFORE SWALLOWING. Food should basically be liquid before you swallow.

17 DO NOT DRINK WHILE EATING. Liquids dilute your digestive enzymes.

18 HYDRATION. Drinking half your body weight in ounces helps out the kidneys and liver. When your kidneys are dehydrated, the liver stops its main jobs and helps out the kidneys. When you are well hydrated, the liver can focus on burning fat. Be nice to your liver, people!

19 DECREASE STRESS. If you hate your job, it is time to find a new one that will embrace this new lifestyle, too. I had one client quit his job to become a fitness instructor. Man, he looks like a new person!

Exercise is a stressor too. Do not plan on running a marathon in the middle of a divorce or if a death occurred in the family. You only have so much stress hormone produced each day. During a stressful time in your life, yoga is a better fit.

Decrease stressful eating situations. This is also why I hate it when clients have business lunch meetings. It really messes with digestion.

Evaluate relationships that are causing too much stress. Are some people in your life toxic and trying to demolish your health goals? It may be time to find more supportive people in your life.

20 ADD CINNAMON TO MEALS. Cinnamon promotes healthy digestion and metabolism and has recently been studied for its effects on blood sugar and cholesterol levels.

21 ADD HERBS AND SPICES TO YOUR MEALS. I love to hide herbs in my meatloaf, meatballs, chili, and spaghetti sauce.

22 CHANGE YOUR SKIN CARE AND TOPICAL PRODUCTS. The liver can become congested from not only the foods you eat, but all of the make-up and soaps you use on your skin! I had one client who had her liver enzymes go back to normal once she ditched all of the lotions and make-up products she was using! Remember the health and fitness magazines I referred to in chapter 2 on pure protein and fat? Well, I despise them for a whole other reason. I realized that the entire magazines are filled with nothing but advertisements, even the articles. I flipped through one magazine's ten-page spread on its top choices for make-up and lotions. If the magazine writers really knew what happened to your body when you put those toxic chemicals on your skin, they wouldn't be pushing fake tanners and toxic sun screens.

Everything you put onto your skin gets shuttled into your bloodstream just as if you ate it. Think I'm crazy? There is a huge pharmaceutical industry that uses topical patches and lotions for medical use. Many times, the topical medications are absorbed better than oral ones. So it would be silly to dismiss the effects of all of the toxic junk we apply daily.

Stop and think about everything going on your skin and gums:

- Toothpaste and/or mouthwash
- Shampoo and/or conditioner
- Soaps
- Lotions
- Make-up
- Deodorant

I am one to enjoy wearing a light perfume. I love Elizabeth Arden's Green Tea, but dare I put it on my skin? Absolutely not! I put it on my clothes. I suggest you start doing the same.

23 DRINK REVERSE OSMOSIS WATER AND CHOOSE ORGANIC FOODS. Get rid of all the fluoride and chlorine in your body. Many fruits, veggies, and other crops in the US are sprayed with cryolite, which is a pesticide that contains a high amount of energy-zapping fluoride. Today, Americans consume four times the amount of fluoride than we did in 1940, which was when it was added to drinking water to prevent cavities. It is found in many commercial products like soup, soda, and many other foods like black tea. Even the Center for Disease Control (CDC) has expressed concern that over two hundred million Americans are exposed to extreme levels of fluoride. As well, all of this is wreaking havoc on our thyroid.

24 ACTIVATE BROWN FAT. There are two types of fat in the body:

1. White adipose tissue (WAT) is what we normally refer to as "body fat." We want to burn white fat. Brown fat is beneficial because it helps burn calories and burns the unhealthy WAT.

2. Brown adipose tissue (BAT) is composed of iron-containing mitochondria (the "powerhouse" of cells), which is best known for creating ATP (energy). More mitochondria = more energy! BAT helps use excess calories for heat. If you use the techniques shown in this book, you can use BAT to your advantage so excess calories aren't stored as WAT (which ends up as undesired belly fat). Cold stimulates BAT to burn excess fat and glucose for energy.

Brown Fat Tips

1. Use ice packs on the back or neck for 30–60 minutes while relaxing at night, when insulin levels are higher and more sensitive.

2. Soak your feet in cold water at night or right away in morning when you first wake up. This will stimulate heat throughout the day.

3. Suck on ice cubes throughout the day. I use mini–ice cubes and sweeten the ice with Capella's Pina Colada drops.

4. Have a "snow cone" for dessert with flavored stevia drops like Root Beer.

5. Take a very cold shower upon waking.

6. Lower the temperature in your house by five degrees.

The following examples can help you burn more calories:

Drinking ice water = burn 60 calories

Sucking on six flavored ice cubes = burn 60 calories

Soaking feet in ice water for 5 minutes = burn 90 calories

Placing ice packs on body for 30 minutes = burn 100 calories

Lowering house temperature by five degrees = burn 100 calories per day

Taking a three minute shower at 75°F = burn 120 calories

25 START OIL PULLING. I know that this sounds crazy, but swishing coconut oil in your mouth for a few minutes a day is an extremely healthy and tasty daily regime that I like to practice. It is extremely easy too. Place a tablespoon of coconut oil in your mouth and swish it around as if it were mouthwash (if it is solid, it will melt in your mouth). Just like brushing your teeth, when you do something for sixteen days in a row it becomes a habit! My suggestion is to toss out your mouthwash filled with chemicals and replace it with a jar of coconut oil.

Here are some of the reasons why you should start "oil pulling" today:

1. It removes bacteria, parasites, and toxins that live in your lymph system. Coconut oil in particular has antimicrobial, anti-inflammatory, and enzymatic properties, which is why I suggest pulling with coconut oil over other oils. It helps kill Streptococcus mutans, an acid-producing bacterium that is a major cause of tooth decay. It also clears up candida, which can cause thrush.

2. It relieves congestion and mucus in your sinuses and throat.

3. Coconut oil remineralizes teeth and strengthens gums.

4. It clears up skin issues like psoriasis because the "pulling" detoxes toxins, which boosts the immune system.

Coconut oil serves several purposes. Its butyric acid is known to increase T3 uptake in the glial cells. It also has a general pro-thyroid action. For example, by diluting and displacing antithyroid unsaturated oils, its short- and medium-chain fatty acids sustain blood sugar and have anti-allergic actions. It also protects mitochondria against stress injury. So if you are like me, get yourself a gallon since you will be using it so much — this will help save you money.

2 6 BEWARE OF CARBONATED BEVERAGES. Have you ever noticed that if you drink champagne (as opposed to wine), you get tipsier faster? Or if you drink vodka with a carbonated soda (as opposed to vodka mixed with juice) you also get tipsier faster? Carbonation increases absorption. The reason I bring up alcohol is not because I want you to start drinking your liquor without carbonation, but because you aren't going to waste your calories and sugar on alcohol anyway, right? I bring this up because when you drink carbonated water, such as a soda from your soda streamer, you increase the rate of absorption.[58]

Remember, I do not recommend drinking while eating because it dilutes your digestive enzymes, but if you do and you choose a carbonated beverage, you may be doing more harm than you think. If you consume a carbonated beverage while eating, especially if you have gone through gastric bypass surgery or have had a gastric sleeve put in, the carbonation forces food through a pouch created by the gastric sleeve, decreasing the time food stays in the pouch, which causes less satiety and an increased desire for food.

Food forced through the pouch by carbonation can also significantly increase the size of the opening between the pouch and intestines, an area called the stoma. An enlarged stoma or pouch permits and encourages you to eat more food in order to feel satiated. In this way, consuming carbonated beverages, even if the drinks are diet or calorie free, may inhibit your weight loss goals.

Chapter 10

Recipes

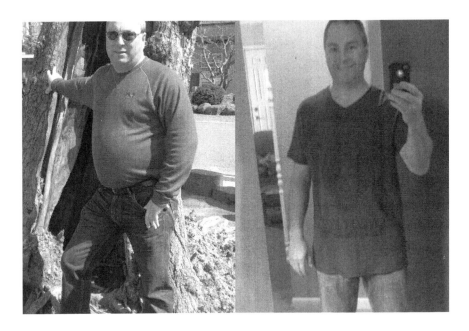

After years of not watching what I ate, I finally found myself at my highest weight ever at age 49. I was also going through some tough times in my life; I was going through a divorce, not by my choice. I was at a crossroads in my life: Being single now after fifteen years of marriage, a father to two wonderful boys, and trying to juggle work amongst all of that. I started talking with a friend who encouraged me to get back on my feet again, telling me that it's easy to lose the weight, which in turn will make you feel good about yourself and give you energy.

I figured, "Why not? What do I have to lose, besides the weight?" It took a very short time to get used to eating differently; it much was easier than I expected. When I started eating low-carb and high-fat and took out the grains, I saw results immediately. I saw the weight come off very quickly and it wasn't hard at all. As a single dad, I am able to eat my eggs for breakfast, take a lunch that I pack each day, and still have a homemade meal at night. I really enjoy the foods I eat. It's not hard at all to take the time to make sure what goes in the mouth is made at home (not from a box) and packing a lunch is so easy. I sometimes use a crock pot to cook meats or soups that are ready to go when I walk in the door after a long day of work.

I have lost approximately 40 pounds and am eating better than ever. I have a more satisfied digestive system as well, not dealing with gas and diarrhea like I used to. I am slowly learning as I go, taking baby steps to eliminate one thing at a time. I really don't miss the way I used to eat, especially after hearing so many people comment on how "skinny" I look. It makes me feel good about myself and I am once again getting some self-confidence back. Thank you Maria for all you do.

—Bill

The only veggies allowed when trying to become keto-adapted are: red leaf lettuce, cabbage, celery, zucchini and cucumbers. I know this sounds crazy, but even non-starchy vegetables may hold you back while trying to become keto-adapted. I used to be more passive in my office and tell clients to take "baby steps" but not anymore. People want results. Rip that band-aid off! Whether you are dealing with inflammation showing externally where people can see it (weight gain, acne, eczema, and rosacea) or internally (heart disease, joint pain, nerve damage, high blood sugar), the faster you can get to be keto-adapted the better. Once adapted or near your weight loss and healing goals, you can begin to re-introduce other low starch veggies. When in maintenance, you can find your bodies threshold for carbs by introducing psyllium breads and nut flours and monitoring your weight (typically 30-50 grams of total carbs per day).

SIDE DISHES

BONE BROTH

This recipe is for a very large amount. I suggest that if you are going to the trouble of making it, do a huge batch, and then store any extra in the freezer in individual packages. Bone broth has many health and healing benefits.

INGREDIENTS:

2 oz roasted garlic

10 oz roasted organic red onions

1 oz coconut oil

4.5 gallons filtered water

22 oz tomato paste (from glass jar)

2 pounds organic chicken backbones

16 oz organic tomato pulp

6 oz Celtic sea salt

1 oz fresh ground black pepper

Optional:

2 to 4 oz rosemary (enhances calcium extraction)

4 oz organic cilantro with stems (good source of potassium, iron, calcium, magnesium, and vitamin A and K)

4 oz organic oregano (good source of potassium, iron, calcium, magnesium, and vitamin C)

DIRECTIONS:

1   In a huge pot, roast onions and garlic in oil for 15 to 20 minutes. Add the rest of the ingredients to the pot.

2   Let simmer over low heat for 2 to 3 days. The longer you cook it, the more nutrients are extracted from the bones, and the darker and thicker the broth will be. Makes 5 gallons.

> **HEALTH TIP:** Once your kimchi or fermented veggies are gone, drink the liquid they are stored in. I suggest at least ¼ cup of the fermented liquid about 15 minutes before meals to help with digestion, acid reflux, and eliminate sugar cravings.

KIMCHI

Kimchi is a traditional Korean dish of fermented vegetables, the most common of which are napa cabbage and daikon radish. In addition to being served as a side dish, my friend Julie suggested I try it over my eggs at breakfast. Wow! It is awesome! You can also use it as a sauce for my "healthified" braised short ribs.

INGREDIENTS:

1 napa cabbage (2 pounds)

½ cup Celtic sea salt

12 cups cold filtered water (add more as needed)

8 oz daikon radish, peeled and cut into 2-inch matchsticks

4 medium scallions, ends trimmed and cut into 1-inch pieces (use all parts)

⅓ cup Korean red pepper powder

¼ cup fish sauce (don't skip this, it provides "umami")

¼ cup peeled and minced fresh ginger

1 tbsp minced garlic cloves

2 tsp Korean salted shrimp, minced

DIRECTIONS:

1   Cut the cabbage in half lengthwise, then crosswise into 2-inch pieces, discarding the root end. Place in a large bowl, sprinkle with salt, and toss with your hands until the cabbage is coated.

2   Add enough cold water to cover it (about 12 cups), making sure the cabbage is covered with water. Cover with a baking sheet and let sit at room temperature for at least 12 hours and up to 24 hours.

3   Place a colander in the sink, drain the cabbage, and rinse with cold water. Gently squeeze out the excess liquid and transfer to a medium-sized bowl. Set it aside.

4   Place the remaining ingredients in a large bowl and stir to combine. Add the cabbage and toss with your hands until evenly combined and the cabbage is thoroughly coated with the mixture.

5   Pack the mixture tightly into a clean 2-quart or 2-liter glass jar with a tight-fitting lid and seal the jar. Let sit in a cool, dark place for 24 hours (the mixture may bubble).

6   Open the jar to let the gases escape, then reseal and refrigerate at least 48 hours before eating (kimchi is best after fermenting about 1 week). Refrigerate for up to 1 month. Makes 16 servings

NUTRITIONAL COMPARISON (PER SERVING)

"HEALTHIFIED" KIMCHI = 15 CALORIES, 0G FAT, 1G PROTEIN, 2G CARBS, 0 FIBER (0% FAT, 35% PROTEIN, 65% CARBS)

BACON CHEDDAR DEVILED EGGS

INGREDIENTS:

12 eggs

½ cup avocado, mashed until smooth

4 slices bacon

2 tbsp cheddar cheese, shredded (if not dairy sensitive)

1 tbsp mustard

DIRECTIONS:

1   Place eggs in a saucepan and cover with cold water. Bring water to a boil then immediately remove from heat. Cover and let eggs stand in hot water for 10 to 12 minutes. Remove from hot water and rinse eggs under cold running water to cool.

2   Meanwhile, place bacon in a large, deep skillet. Cook over medium-high heat until evenly brown. Crumble and set aside. Peel the hard-cooked eggs, and cut in half lengthwise. Remove yolks and place them in a small bowl. Mash egg yolks with avocado, crumbled bacon, and cheese. Stir in mustard. Fill egg white halves with the yolk mixture and refrigerate until serving. Makes 12 servings.

NUTRITIONAL COMPARISON (PER SERVING)

"HEALTHIFIED" DEVILED EGGS = 107 CALORIES, 8.2G FAT, 7.5G PROTEIN, 0.7G CARBS, 0.6G FIBER (69% FAT, 28% PROTEIN, 3% CARBS)

SUPER SALAD DRESSING

INGREDIENTS:

½ cup liquid MCT oil

4 tbsp coconut vinegar

½ tsp stevia glycerite

1 tsp Celtic sea salt

½ tsp fresh ground pepper

½ tsp fish sauce

DIRECTIONS:

1   Place all ingredients into a salad jar and shake vigorously. Use for cole-slaw or drizzle on your salad greens. Makes 10 servings.

NUTRITIONAL COMPARISON (PER SERVING)

STORE BOUGHT ASIAN DRESSING = 140 CALORIES, 12G FAT, 0G PROTEIN, 6G CARBS, 0 FIBER

"HEALTHIFIED" ASIAN DRESSING = 96 CALORIES, 11.2G FAT, 0G PROTEIN, 0.1 CARBS, 0 FIBER (99% FAT, 0% PROTEIN, <1% CARBS)

BACONAISE

INGREDIENTS:

2 egg yolks

1 tsp mustard

3 tsp lemon juice

1 cup liquid bacon fat or rendered lard (or ½ cup MCT oil and ½ cup expeller pressed coconut oil)

TIP: If you use expeller pressed coconut oil in place of the bacon fat, don't worry about an overwhelming coconut flavor — this type of coconut oil does not have a coconut taste.

DIRECTIONS:

1   Place the yolks, mustard, and 1 tsp of the lemon juice in a food processor or blender and combine until smooth. Start blending on low (or whisking vigorously if you are doing it by hand) while dripping the oil

very slowly (drop by drop in the beginning). TIP: You're creating an emulsion and if you put too much oil in at once, it will separate and will be very hard to save.

2   As you add more oil, the emulsion will form and the mayonnaise will start to thicken. You can pour the oil faster at this point.

3   When all the oil has been added and the mayonnaise is thick, add the rest of the lemon juice and taste your creation. You can season to taste with salt and pepper. Makes 22 servings.

NUTRITIONAL COMPARISON (PER SERVING)
STORE BOUGHT MAYO = 90 CALORIES, 10G FAT, 0G PROTEIN, 0G CARBS, 0 FIBER
"HEALTHIFIED" MAYO = 104 CALORIES, 11G FAT, 0G PROTEIN, 0G CARBS, 0 FIBER (100% FAT, 0% PROTEIN, 0% CARBS)

FOIS GRAS

Sautéing duck foie gras is not hard to do, but be careful; otherwise, you'll end up with a puddle of very expensive melted fat.

INGREDIENTS:
½ pound piece raw Grade A duck foie gras at room temperature, cleaned and deveined
Celtic sea salt and pepper to taste
2 tsp coconut oil
2 tbsp coconut or balsamic vinegar

DIRECTIONS:

1   After deveining, cut the foie gras crosswise into ½-inch-thick pieces, then season with salt and pepper.

2   Heat 1 teaspoon of oil in a 10-inch heavy skillet over moderately high heat until hot (but not smoking).

3   Sauté half the foie gras until golden, 45 to 60 seconds on each side (it will be pink inside). Quickly transfer to a paper towel in order to drain

and discard fat in skillet. Sauté the rest of the foie gras the same way, then discard all but 1 tablespoon of remaining fat in skillet.

4   Add 2 tablespoons of vinegar to remaining oil and bring to a boil. Simmer until sauce is reduced by half. Serve foie gras with sauce. Makes 4 servings.

NUTRITIONAL COMPARISON (PER SERVING)

"HEALTHIFIED" FOIS GRAS = 292 CALORIES, 28G FAT, 7G PROTEIN, 3G CARBS, 1.2G FIBER (86% FAT, 10% PROTEIN, 4% CARBS)

PROTEIN POPOVERS

INGREDIENTS:
1 cup Jay Robb's unflavored whey protein (or vanilla for a sweet popover)

4 tbsp coconut oil, melted (plus extra for greasing)

2 cups unflavored almond milk

4 eggs

½ tsp Celtic sea salt

DIRECTIONS:

1   Preheat the oven to 425 degrees F. Grease popover tins with coconut oil. Place the tins in the hot oven for about 8 minutes. Meanwhile, in a medium-sized bowl blend together the whey, almond milk, eggs, and salt.

2   Carefully remove hot tins from oven. Dollop 1 tsp of coconut oil into each hot tin and pour the batter in until 2/3 full. Bake for 15 minutes. Leave the oven closed and reduce heat to 325 degrees F to bake for an additional 10 to 12 minutes. Makes 12 servings.

NUTRITIONAL COMPARISON (PER POPOVER)

TRADITIONAL POPOVER = 152 CALORIES, 7 G FAT, 2 G PROTEIN, 20 CARBS, 0 FIBER

"HEALTHIFIED" POPOVER = 106 CALORIES, 7 G FAT, 10 G PROTEIN, 1.2 CARBS, 0 FIBER (60% FAT, 37% PROTEIN, 3% CARBS)

BREAKFAST IDEAS

EGGS BENEDICT ON PROTEIN BUN

INGREDIENTS:

6 large egg yolks

¼ cup lemon juice

2 tbsp Dijon mustard

1 ½ cups melted organic butter (or melted bacon fat or duck fat)

¼ tsp Celtic sea salt (or more to taste)

1/8 tsp freshly ground black pepper

PROTEIN BUN

3 eggs, separated

½ cup Jay Robb's unflavored egg white protein (or whey protein)

½ tsp fresh dill or other herb of your choice

ADDITIONS

6 ham (or prosciutto) slices

12 large eggs

DIRECTIONS:

1   **To make the buns:** Preheat the oven to 325 degrees F.

2   Separate the eggs (save the yolks in another bowl), and whip the whites for a few minutes until very stiff (I use a stand mixer on high for a few minutes).

3   Gently mix the protein powder and herbs into the egg whites.

4   Slowly fold the egg yolks into the whites, making sure the whites don't "fall" (collapse back into liquid).

5   Grease a cookie sheet with coconut oil spray and place mounds of the egg white mixture about the size of a hamburger bun onto the sheet.

6   Bake for 40 to 45 minutes or until golden brown.

7   Let completely cool before cutting or the buns will "fall."

8   **To make hollandaise sauce:** In the bottom of a double boiler or in a medium-sized saucepan, bring 1 inch of water to a simmer over high heat. Adjust heat to maintain simmer. Put egg yolks, lemon juice, and mustard in top section of double boiler or in a round-bottomed medium bowl and set over simmering water. Whisk yolk mixture to blend.

9   Whisking constantly, add butter to the yolk mixture in a slow, steady stream (it should take about 90 seconds). Cook sauce, whisking, until it reaches 140 degrees F (using a candy thermometer), then adjust heat to maintain temperature (remove from simmering water if necessary). Add salt, pepper, and cayenne and continue whisking until thick (it will take about 3 minutes). Adjust seasonings to taste. Remove from stove and set aside.

10 Put 2 bun halves on each plate and top with ham.

11 **To poach eggs:** Bring 1 inch water to boil in a 12-inch-wide pan. Lower heat so that small bubbles form on the bottom of the pan and break to the surface only occasionally. Crack eggs into water one at a time, holding shells close to the water's surface and letting eggs slide out gently. Poach eggs in 2 batches to keep them from crowding for 3 to 4 minutes for soft-cooked eggs. Lift eggs out with a slotted spoon, pat dry with a paper towel, and place 1 egg on each slice of ham.

12 Top each egg with 2 to 3 tbsp of hollandaise sauce. Serve hot. Makes 6 servings.

NUTRITIONAL COMPARISON (PER POPOVER)

TRADITIONAL EGGS BENEDICT = 1020 CALORIES, 57G FAT, 43G PROTEIN, 80G CARBS, 6G FIBER

"HEALTHIFIED" EGGS BENEDICT = 716 CALORIES, 65.4G FAT, 29.4G PROTEIN, 3.5G CARBS, 0.6G FIBER (82% FAT, 16% PROTEIN, 2% CARBS)

HUEVOS RANCHEROS

TORTILLAS

Coconut oil/ghee/butter (for frying)

3 egg, separated

¼ cup Jay Robb's unflavored egg white protein or whey protein

2 tbsp cream cheese, very soft (or reserved egg yolks if dairy allergy)

1 tsp onion powder

Optional: 1 tsp Mexican spices

TOPPING IDEAS

½ cup browned grass fed beef (or my chili recipe)

fried eggs, avocado, salsa, green onions, peppers

DIRECTIONS:

1   Place the egg whites (can't have yolks at all or it won't work) in a bowl and whip with a hand mixer or stand mixer until whites are very stiff.

2   Slowly add in the unflavored protein powder and spices.

3   Then gently stir in the cream cheese or yolks.

4   Heat oil in a small skillet over medium-high heat.

5   Fry tortilla dough one at a time until firm, but not crisp.

6   Once crisp, remove tortillas and place onto paper towels to drain any excess oil.

7   Meanwhile, prepare the beef and other desired toppings.

8   Optional: When tortillas are done, fry eggs over easy in the skillet.

9   Place tortillas onto plates, and spread a layer of meat on them.

10 Top with your desired toppings. I love my chili, a fried egg, crumbled bacon, avocado, and salsa. Makes 4 servings.

NUTRITIONAL COMPARISON (PER SERVING)

TRADITIONAL DISH = 495 CALORIES, 20G FAT, 21G PROTEIN, 24.2G CARBS, 5.2G FIBER

"HEALTHIFIED" DISH = 329 CALORIES, 24G FAT, 24G PROTEIN, 5.7G CARBS, 3.5G FIBER (66% FAT, 29% PROTEIN, 6% CARBS)

BREAKFAST CHILI

2 pounds grass fed ground beef

1 pound ground liver or spicy Italian sausage

4 cups tomato sauce (preferably homemade organic or from a glass jar)

½ yellow onion, chopped

3 stalks of celery, chopped

1 green bell pepper, seeded and chopped

1 red bell pepper, seeded and chopped

2 green chili peppers, seeded and chopped

2 slices of bacon

1 cup organic beef broth

¼ cup chili powder

1 tbsp minced garlic

3 tbsp fresh oregano

2 tsp ground cumin

3 tbsp fresh basil

1 tsp Celtic sea salt

1 tsp ground black pepper

1 tsp cayenne pepper

1 tsp paprika

TOPPINGS:

fried eggs

avocado, cubed into 1 cm chunks

cooked bacon, crumbled

1   Heat a large stock pot over medium-high heat.

2   Crumble the ground beef, bacon and, sausage into the hot pan, and cook until evenly browned. Drain any excess grease.

3   Pour in the tomato sauce. Add the onion, celery, green and red bell peppers, chili peppers, and broth. Season with chili powder, garlic, oregano, cumin, basil, salt, pepper, cayenne, and paprika. Stir to blend, then cover and simmer over low heat for at least 2 hours, stirring occasionally.

4   After 2 hours, taste. If necessary, add salt, pepper, and chili powder. The longer the chili simmers, the better it will taste.

5   Remove from heat and serve, or refrigerate and serve the next day. Top with avocado slices, a fried egg, and bacon crumble. Makes 12 servings.

NUTRITIONAL COMPARISON (PER SERVING)

TRADITIONAL CHILI = 293 CALORIES, 7.9G FAT, 18G PROTEIN, 37G CARBS, 8G FIBER (WITHOUT FRIED EGG, AVOCADO AND BACON)

"HEALTHIFIED" CHILI = 485 CALORIES, 30.3G FAT, 35.7G PROTEIN, 10G CARBS, 5G FIBER (58% FAT, 30% PROTEIN, 10% CARBS) (WITH EGG, AVOCADO AND BACON)

CRUSTLESS SMOKED SALMON QUICHE

INGREDIENTS:

1 cup leeks, slicing both white and light green parts

½ cup red pepper, chopped

4 oz raw mushrooms

2 tbsp fresh thyme, chopped fine

6 oz smoked salmon

4 eggs

1 ½ cup unsweetened and unflavored almond milk

¾ cup crumbled goat cheese

1 tsp dry mustard

1 tsp paprika

½ tsp Celtic sea salt

½ tsp fresh ground pepper

¼ tsp cayenne pepper (or add to desired heat)

DIRECTIONS:

1   Preheat oven to 375 degrees F. Sauté leeks in a little coconut oil. When they begin to soften, add mushrooms. After a minute or two, add the peppers. Add a little salt and cook for 3 to 4 minutes. Just before taking off heat, add the fresh thyme.

2   Meanwhile, crumble salmon into a 9-inch pie plate. Cover with sautéed vegetables and sprinkle with cheese.

3   In a separate bowl, blend eggs, milk, mustard, paprika, salt, pepper, and cayenne. You can use an eggbeater or whisk, but a blender works really well. Pour the egg mixture over the rest of the ingredients. Bake for 35 to 50 minutes.

4   Check the quiche after 30 minutes. If it's getting too brown but the middle is too liquid, cover with foil. When done, the center will still be a bit loose.

5   Take quiche out of the oven or the rest will overcook. In 5 minutes, the center will have finished cooking from the heat of the surrounding quiche. Makes 4 servings.

NUTRITIONAL COMPARISON (PER SERVING)

TRADITIONAL QUICHE = 716 CALORIES, 47G FAT, 22G PROTEIN, 42G CARBS, 3G FIBER

"HEALTHIFIED" QUICHE = 363 CALORIES, 25G FAT, 27G PROTEIN, 8G CARBS, 2G FIBER (62% FAT, 30% PROTEIN, 8% CARBS)

LUNCH AND DINNERS
Keto Niçoise Salad

INGREDIENTS:

DRESSING

½ cup lemon juice

¾ cup MCT oil

1 medium shallot, minced

1 tbsp minced fresh thyme leaves

2 tbsp minced fresh basil leaves

2 tsp minced fresh oregano leaves

1 tsp Dijon mustard

½ tsp Celtic sea salt

¼ tsp freshly ground black pepper

SALAD

2 to 3 cans of tuna (or 2 seared tuna steaks, 8 oz each)

6 hard boiled eggs, peeled and quartered

1 avocado, peeled and sliced into chunks

2 heads of red leaf lettuce, washed and torn into bite-sized pieces

3 small tomatoes, sliced

8 oz green beans, stem ends trimmed and each bean halved crosswise

¼ cup olives

2 tbsp capers, rinsed

Optional:

1 can or more of anchovies

DIRECTIONS:

1   If using tuna steaks, marinate in MCT oil for an hour. Heat a grill or large skillet on medium-high heat. Cook the steaks 1 to 3 minutes on each side until seared or until desired color.

2   To make the dressing, whisk lemon juice, oil, shallot, thyme, basil, oregano, and mustard in medium bowl. Season to taste with salt and pepper, then set aside.

3 Toss lettuce with ¼ cup dressing in large bowl until coated. Arrange lettuce on a serving platter. Coat the tuna with dressing. Mound tuna in center of lettuce.

4 Bring a pot of water to boil, then add a tablespoon of salt and the green beans. Cook until tender, but crisp, for 3 to 5 minutes. Drain beans and rinse with very cold water.

5 Dry beans well and toss with 3 tablespoons dressing (salt and pepper to taste). Arrange beans in a mound at edge of lettuce bed.

6 Place the hard boiled eggs, olives, and anchovies (if using) in mounds on the lettuce bed. Drizzle eggs with remaining 2 tablespoons of dressing, then sprinkle entire salad with capers (if using). Serve immediately. Makes 6 servings.

NUTRITIONAL COMPARISON (PER SERVING)

TRADITIONAL NIÇOISE = 520 CALORIES, 38G FAT, 24.5G PROTEIN, 25.2G CARBS, 4.8G FIBER

HEALTHIFIED NIÇOISE = 499 CALORIES, 42G FAT, 23.5G PROTEIN, 9G CARBS, 4.8G FIBER (76% FAT, 18% PROTEIN, 6% CARBS)

BLT

INGREDIENTS:

2 slices protein bread

2 tbsp baconaise mayo (see baconaise recipe)

2 slices red leaf lettuce

1 slice tomato

2 slices bacon, cooked

DIRECTIONS:

1 Slice the protein bread, spread with baconaise, top with lettuce, tomato and bacon. Makes 1 serving.

NUTRITIONAL COMPARISON (PER SERVING)

TRADITIONAL BLT = 450 CALORIES, 18G FAT, 18G PROTEIN, 53G CARBS, 2G FIBER

"HEALTHIFIED" BLT = 446 CALORIES, 40G FAT, 19G PROTEIN, 9G CARBS, 4G FIBER (80% FAT, 16% PROTEIN, 7% CARBS)

SEAFOOD AVOCADO SALAD

1 pound seafood (shrimp, real crab, or any firm fish will work well)

2 avocados, peeled and cubed

2 tomatoes, cubed

4 to 6 green onions, minced

Juice of 1 lime or lemon

1 tbsp macadamia nut or avocado oil

A handful of fresh cilantro, chopped

A pinch of Celtic sea salt and fresh pepper

DIRECTIONS:

1   Coat all the ingredients thoroughly with lime juice because the avocado will turn brown without it. Assemble the salad into a bowl.

2   Cover with Saran Wrap right on top of the salad to help prevent oxygen from getting to your lovely little avocado bits. This stuff is really good on a bed of lettuce. Makes 4 servings.

NUTRITIONAL COMPARISON (PER SERVING)

"HEALTHIFIED" SALAD = 380 CALORIES, 27G FAT, 28G PROTEIN, 6G CARBS, 6G FIBER (64% FAT, 29% PROTEIN, 6% CARBS)

MCT Pesto

Have you ever heard of Beyonce's Maple Syrup Diet cleanse? It is just water, lemon juice, cayenne, and maple syrup. I like the lemon and the cayenne part of the cleanse, but the maple syrup? No, no, no! Switch that out with coconut oil, and you now have a fat burning meal that won't cause you to be "hangry" (hungry and angry).

As I thought about people actually doing the crazy maple syrup diet, I thought, hmm, I can make a recipe that will really stimulate fat burning. So I made this pesto, which includes lime juice for cleansing, coconut oil for ketones, basil for phytonutrients (herbs have *way* more vitamins and minerals than any fruit or vegetable has), and cayenne pepper for calorie burning. Spicy peppers cause the body temperature to rise. When the body temperature rises, it needs to be cooled; you burn extra calories when the body is forced to go through a cooling process. The downside of this trick is when you become accustomed to spicy foods, it takes more spice to raise your body temperature. You basically build up a tolerance.

So if you like pesto sauce, you must try this great "pure protein and fat" dinner I had last night with kelp noodles. If you cook the kelp noodles in a slow cooker on low for eight hours with the pesto, the noodles get really soft and suck up that pesto goodness! But do not buy pre-made pesto — make your own! Store bought pesto often has soybean oil. Even if it is made with olive oil, you can increase your level of fat burning if you make it with coconut oil or MCT oil! Olive oil is a long-chain triglyceride; I always use liquid MCT oil in my recipes and salad dressings. Medium-chain triglycerides (MCTs) are different than long-chain triglycerides. MCTs are absorbed more like carbohydrates and are used and burned quickly by the body. They are not stored in the fat cells, and any extra are converted into ketones. (I used protein bread to make garlic bread with my meal to keep it "pure protein and fat.")

INGREDIENTS:
1 package kelp noodles

2 cups basil (compacted/pushed down)

¼ cup melted coconut oil (can substitute with macadamia nut oil)

4 tbsp MCT oil (can substitute with coconut oil)

¼ cup walnuts

3 garlic cloves

3 tbsp fresh red chili (add more or less, depending on desired heat)

2 tbsp lime juice (optional)

⅓ tsp Celtic sea salt

¼ tsp freshly ground pepper

¼ cup freshly grated Parmesan cheese (if not dairy sensitive)

1   Place basil, oil, walnuts, garlic, chilis, lime juice, salt, and pepper into a food processor and blend until smooth.

2   Place the kelp noodles with the pesto into a 4-quart slow cooker on low for 6 to 8 hours. The kelp noodles will get very soft.

3   Serve with protein bread. To make "garlic bread," brush protein bread with macadamia nut oil and rub roasted garlic on it, then cook in the oven at 400 degrees F for 3 to 6 minutes or until toasted. Makes 4 servings.

NUTRITIONAL COMPARISON (PER SERVING)

TRADITIONAL PESTO NOODLES =
    628 CALORIES, 35.4G FAT, 14G PROTEIN, 65.3G CARBS, 1.3G FIBER

"HEALTHIFIED" PESTO NOODLES =
    300 CALORIES, 32G FAT, 2G PROTEIN, 3G CARBS, 1.3G FIBER
    (95% FAT, 2% PROTEIN, 3% CARBS)

SUPER HEALTHY SPAGHETTI BOLOGNAISE

Health Tip: A great protein and fat source for a keto-adapted diet is organic organ meat, which is one of the only natural sources of K2 (different from K1). K1 is a blood clotter, whereas K2 helps reverse artery calcification and Alzheimer's, increases fertility, and has anti-aging properties as well as many other healing properties. I'm not a fan of organ meat's taste (and I don't expect you to be either), so I hide it in foods like this meatloaf!

Are you concerned that your kids or spouse don't get enough fruits and veggies like you think they should? Eating fresh herbs will fill your body with more vitamins and minerals than any sugary fruit will.

INGREDIENTS:

1 tbsp coconut oil

2 packages kelp noodles

4 oz bacon or pancetta, diced

½ cup chopped yellow onions

¾ cup diced celery

1 tbsp minced garlic

1 tsp Celtic sea salt

½ tsp ground black pepper

2 bay leaves

¼ cup fresh parsley

3 tbsp fresh thyme

3 tbsp fresh oregano

½ tsp ground cinnamon

½ tsp ground nutmeg

1 pound grass fed ground beef

½ pound organic pork sausage, casings removed, or ground pork

½ pound ground organic liver

2 cups tomato sauce (from glass jar)

4 cups crushed tomatoes and their juice

1 cup organic beef (or chicken stock or broth)

½ tsp stevia glycerite (if desired for a little sweetness)

Optional (if not dairy sensitive):

¼ cup organic heavy cream

2 tbsp organic butter

1 cup freshly grated Parmesan

DIRECTIONS:

1   Rinse and drain the kelp noodles. Place the kelp noodles with water in a 6-quart slow cooker on low for 2 to 6 hours or until desired softness. Remove from slow cooker and drain water. Set aside to top with bolognaise sauce later.

2   While the kelp noodles cook, make the bolognaise. In a large pot, heat the coconut oil over medium-high heat.

3   Add the bacon. Cook for 4 to 5 minutes, stirring, until browned and the fat is rendered.

4   Add the onions and celery. Cook for 4 to 5 minutes, stirring, until soft.

5   Add the garlic, salt, pepper, bay leaves, thyme, oregano, cinnamon, and nutmeg. Cook for 30 seconds, stirring.

6   Turn heat to low, then add the beef, pork, and liver. Cook for about 7 minutes, stirring, until meat is no longer pink.

7   Add the tomato sauce and cook for 1 to 2 minutes, stirring.

8   Deglaze the pan and remove any browned bits sticking to the bottom of the pan, and until half of the liquid is evaporated, about 2 minutes.

9   Add the tomatoes and their juices, broth (and stevia if using) and bring to a boil.

10 Reduce the heat to medium-low and simmer, stirring occasionally, to keep the sauce from sticking to the bottom of the pan, until the sauce is thickened and flavorful, about 1 ½ hours.

11 If no dairy sensitivity, add cream, butter and stir well, simmer for 2 minutes. Discard the bay leaves and adjust the seasoning, to taste.

12 Remove from the heat and cover to keep warm until ready to serve. Add the reserved kelp noodles. Sprinkle with Parmesan if desired. Makes 12 servings.

NUTRITIONAL COMPARISON (PER SERVING)

TRADITIONAL BOLOGNAISE = 460 CALORIES, 6G FAT, 18G PROTEIN, 92G CARBS, 6G FIBER

"HEALTHIFIED" BOLOGNAISE = 251 CALORIES, 12G FAT, 23G PROTEIN, 13G CARBS, 3G FIBER (43% FAT, 37% PROTEIN, 20% CARBS)

SUPER HEALTHY MEATLOAF

INGREDIENTS:

½ cup yellow onion

2 stalks celery

2 tbsp tallow or coconut oil

4 cloves garlic, crushed

1 pound ground pork

1 pound ground beef

1 pound liver

½ cup tomato sauce (preferably from a glass jar)

¼ cup fresh parsley

3 tbsp fresh basil

3 tbsp fresh oregano

1 tbsp fresh thyme

1 tbsp fresh chives

2 tsp paprika

½ tsp pepper

2 tbsp coconut aminos

3 tbsp coconut vinegar

1 tbsp fish sauce

2 eggs

Optional:

¼ tsp stevia glycerite

DIRECTIONS:

1   Finely chop the onions and celery.

2   Heat tallow or coconut oil in a frying pan over medium-high heat.

3   Add the onion and celery and sauté until soft and starting to brown (about 8 to 10 minutes).

4   Finely chop parsley, basil, oregano, thyme, and chives. Crush garlic. Grind the liver in a food processor or meat grinder (you can always ask your butcher to grind it, also).

5   Combine all of the ingredients in a large bowl. Mix together very thoroughly (I find it easiest to just get my hands in there).

6   Cover and refrigerate for 6 hours or overnight to let the flavors combine.

7   Preheat oven to 350 degrees F. Press meat mixture into a large loaf pan. Place the loaf pan on a cookie sheet in case juices run over. Bake for 1 hour 40 minutes or until internal temperature reaches 160 degrees F.

8   Let it sit for 5 to 10 minutes before serving. The juices are really yummy with some protein garlic bread! Makes 8 servings.

NUTRITIONAL COMPARISON (PER SERVING)

TRADITIONAL MEATLOAF = 460 CALORIES, 22G FAT, 52G PROTEIN, 12G CARBS, 0G FIBER

"HEALTHIFIED" MEATLOAF = 435 CALORIES, 26G FAT, 42G PROTEIN, 7G CARBS, 2G FIBER (54% FAT, 39% PROTEIN, 6% CARBS)

LOBSTER ROLL ON PROTEIN BUN

Lobster is high in cholesterol, which helps the production of hormones like progesterone and testosterone. But since lobster is lower in fat, we add baconaise!

INGREDIENTS:
¼ cup cooked lobster or crab meat

2 tbsp baconaise

1 tsp dill

1 protein bun

DIRECTIONS:

1   In a medium-sized bowl, mix the lobster pieces with baconaise and add dill (or other fresh herbs to desired taste). Place mixture in a split protein bun. Makes 1 serving.

NUTRITIONAL COMPARISON (PER SERVING)

TRADITIONAL ROLL = CALORIES, G FAT, G PROTEIN, G CARBS, G FIBER

"HEALTHIFIED" ROLL = 359 CALORIES, 32G FAT, 17G PROTEIN, 0G CARBS, 0G FIBER
(81% FAT, 19% PROTEIN, 0% CARB)

PAN SEARED SALMON WITH AVOCADO CREAM

INGREDIENTS:

2 large avocados, cut and peeled

3 tbsp freshly squeezed lime juice

3 tbsp coconut oil

1 tbsp minced shallots or green onion

2 tbsp minced parsley

1 tsp Dijon mustard (or to taste)

Pepper and Celtic salt to taste

1 ½ pounds of salmon fillets

Coconut oil or ghee

DIRECTIONS:

1   Put avocado pieces and lime juice into a food processor or blender and pulse until blended. Slowly add oil, still pulsing, until you reach desired consistency of sauce. Add minced shallots (or green onions) and parsley, and pulse just until shallots are combined. Place mixture in a bowl, then add mustard, salt, and pepper to taste.

2   Coat the bottom of a sauté pan with coconut oil on medium-high heat (wait until hot). Season both sides of the salmon fillets with salt and pepper, then carefully lay the salmon into the pan, skin side down.

3   Cook the salmon until the fish flakes easily with a fork (about 3 to 4 minutes per side). Serve salmon with avocado cream sauce. Makes 6 servings.

NUTRITIONAL COMPARISON (PER SERVING)

"HEALTHIFIED" SALMON = 639 CALORIES, 50G FAT, 35G PROTEIN, 12G CARBS, 10G FIBER (71% FAT, 22% PROTEIN, 7% CARBS)

TACO BAR LETTUCE CUPS

INGREDIENTS:
1 head Boston or Romaine lettuce
1 pound organic ground beef
½ cup sliced red and green bell peppers
½ cup sliced onion
Guacamole
Salsa
Organic sour cream (if not dairy sensitive)

FAJITA SEASONING
1 tsp chili powder
¾ tsp paprika
¾ tsp cumin
½ tsp onion powder
½ tsp Celtic sea salt
⅜ tsp garlic powder
Pinch of cayenne

DIRECTIONS:

1 Place beef, peppers, and onions in a medium-sized bowl.

2 Blend fajita seasoning mix with ¼ cup water and pour mixture over the beef and veggies. Stir so that beef and veggies are thoroughly coated.

3 Let marinate for 5 minutes or overnight in fridge.

4 Heat a medium-sized pan to medium-high heat.

5 Pour beef mixture into the pan. Moving mixture around occasionally with a spatula, cook until beef is cooked through and veggies are slightly browned (about 6 minutes).

6 Transfer mixture to a bowl. Serve with lettuce leaves, guacamole, salsa, and sour cream. Enjoy fajita-style by loading up each lettuce "cup" with the mixture and topping with the condiments. Have a "taco bar" night. Makes 6 servings.

NUTRITIONAL COMPARISON (PER SERVING)
TRADITIONAL TACO = 340 CALORIES, 20G FAT, 16G PROTEIN, 24G CARBS, 6G FIBER
"HEALTHIFIED" TACO = 341 CALORIES, 24G FAT, 23G PROTEIN, 8G CARBS, 2G FIBER
  (64% FAT, 27% PROTEIN, 9% CARBS)

EASY KOREAN SHORT RIBS

Note: Most rice vinegars have sugar added to them, so please read labels. The brand STAR's rice vinegar has no sugar.

INGREDIENTS:

½ cup coconut aminos or organic tamari (soy) sauce

⅓ cup Swerve Sweetener (Confectioners Style)

¼ cup rice vinegar

2 cloves garlic, peeled and smashed

1 tbsp grated fresh ginger

½ tsp crushed red pepper

8 grass fed beef short ribs (4 pounds)

1 green cabbage, quartered

½ tsp guar gum (thickener)

1 tbsp sesame oil

4 scallions, thinly sliced

DIRECTIONS:

1   In a 4- to 6-quart slow cooker, combine the coconut aminos (or tamari sauce), natural sweetener, vinegar, garlic, ginger, and red pepper. Add the short ribs, arranging them in a single layer. Lay the cabbage on top.

2   Cook, covered, on low for 7 to 8 hours until the meat is tender and easily pulls away from the bone.

3   Transfer the cabbage and short ribs to plates. With a large spoon or ladle, skim the fat from the cooking liquid and discard, but keep the cooking liquid in the slow cooker. Turn the slow cooker to high.

4   In a small bowl, whisk together the guar gum with 1 tbsp of water until smooth. Whisk into the cooking liquid and cook until thickened (2 to 3 minutes). Stir in the sesame oil. Spoon the sauce over the short ribs and cabbage and sprinkle with the scallions. Makes 8 servings.

NUTRITIONAL COMPARISON (PER SERVING)

TRADITIONAL RIBS = 631 CALORIES, 14G FAT, 21G PROTEIN, 31G CARBS, 2.5G FIBER

"HEALTHIFIED" RIBS = 494 CALORIES, 25G FAT, 66G PROTEIN, 2G CARBS, 0.6G FIBER (45% FAT, 54% PROTEIN, 1.6% CARBS)

"HEALTHIFIED" PAD THAI

INGREDIENTS:

4 cups cabbage, sliced very thin (into noodle-like shapes)

¾ cup Swerve Sweetener (Confectioners Style) or erythritol and 1 tsp stevia glycerite

1 tsp ground cayenne pepper

3 tbsp coconut vinegar or cider vinegar

1 tsp fish sauce

1 tbsp natural SunButter or almond butter

1 tbsp coconut oil

2 cloves garlic, minced

1 tsp ginger, minced

4 large eggs, lightly beaten

½ cup fresh bean sprouts

2 packages Miracle Noodles

1 cup veggie broth

¾ tsp guar gum (thickener)

GARNISHES

½ cup chopped green onion

Fresh cilantro leaves

Mung bean sprouts

CHICKEN OPTION

1 pound chicken thighs with skin

Celtic sea salt and ground black pepper to taste

DIRECTIONS:

1   Slice cabbage into egg noodle widths (very thin). Stir-fry in coconut oil or butter (or you could boil it in water) for 5 to 10 minutes or until very tender. Set aside.

2   Peanut Sauce: Whisk natural sweetener, cayenne pepper, vinegar, fish sauce, and SunButter or almond butter together in a bowl. Coat the inside of a large skillet or wok with oil and place over high heat. Once the temperature reaches high heat, lower the heat under the skillet to

medium-low. Cook and stir garlic and ginger in the skillet until the garlic becomes translucent (1 to 2 minutes).

3   Cook and stir eggs into garlic until mostly cooked (2 to 3 minutes). Pour peanut sauce into the garlic and eggs, and stir to combine. Bring sauce to a simmer, stirring frequently for 5 to 8 more minutes.

4   Stir in Miracle Noodles, the sautéed cabbage noodles, broth, and guar gum into the skillet. Bring to a simmer and cook for about 10 minutes.

5   Place into a serving dish and add desired garnishes before serving. Makes 4 servings.

6   **CHICKEN OPTION**: Heat coconut oil in a skillet. Once hot, place chicken on skillet and cook until the meat is white outside, but still pink inside, for about 3 minutes. Remove chicken and serve over your Pad Thai. Makes 5 servings.

NUTRITIONAL COMPARISON (PER SERVING)

TRADITIONAL PAD THAI = 430 CALORIES, 8G FAT, 20G PROTEIN, 71G CARBS, 3G FIBER

"HEALTHIFIED" PAD THAI = 349 CALORIES, 23G FAT, 28G PROTEIN, 7G CARBS, 2G FIBER
    (60% FAT, 32% PROTEIN, 8% CARBS)

"HEALTHIFIED" PAD THAI (WITHOUT CHICKEN) =
    176 CALORIES, 12G FAT, 11G PROTEIN, 9G CARBS, 2.6G FIBER
    (61% FAT, 22% PROTEIN, 18% CARBS)

"HEALTHIFIED" SHRIMP SCAMPI BAKE

½ cup butter or macadamia nut oil

1 tbsp Dijon mustard

1 tbsp fresh lemon juice

1 tbsp chopped garlic

2 tbsp chopped fresh parsley

1 pound medium raw shrimp (shell on increases flavor)

1 bag kelp noodles

DIRECTIONS:

1   Prepare the kelp noodles according to directions. Set aside in a beautiful serving dish.

2   Preheat oven to 450 degrees F. In a small saucepan over medium heat, combine the butter, mustard, lemon juice, garlic, and parsley. When the butter melts completely, remove from heat.

3   Arrange shrimp in a shallow baking dish. Pour the butter mixture over the shrimp. Bake in preheated oven for 12 to 15 minutes or until the shrimp are pink and opaque.

4   Place baked shrimp and butter sauce over the noodles, peel the shrimp, and enjoy! Serve with "healthified" protein garlic bread. Makes 4 servings.

NUTRITIONAL COMPARISON (PER SERVING)

TRADITIONAL SCAMPI (USING GLUTEN-FREE RICE NOODLES) = 512 CALORIES, 24G FAT, 25G PROTEIN, 45G CARBS, 1G FIBER

"HEALTHIFIED" SCAMPI = 320 CALORIES, 24G FAT, 24G PROTEIN, 1.1G CARB, 0G FIBER (69% FAT, 30% PROTEIN, 1% CARBS)

"HEALTHIFIED" CHICKEN SALAD

INGREDIENTS:

4 cups cubed, smoked chicken meat

1 cup homemade baconaise or organic mayonnaise

1 tsp paprika

1 green onion, chopped

1 cup chopped pecans

1 tsp Celtic sea salt

Ground black pepper to taste

Optional:

Sliced hard boiled eggs

1 cup chopped celery

½ cup minced green pepper

8 protein buns

DIRECTIONS:

1   Clean and cut chicken into thighs, breasts, and wings. Place soaked wood chips in the bottom of your smoker, and place the chicken on the racks. Smoke (outside) for 3 to 4 hours, depending on the manufacturer's directions. At this point you still want to finish cooking it in a preheated oven at 250 degrees F for 30 minutes or until deep golden.

2   In a medium-sized bowl, mix together mayonnaise with paprika and salt. Blend in onion and nuts (and other additions that you prefer, like celery or green pepper). Add chopped poultry and mix well. Season with black pepper to taste. Add sliced hard boiled eggs if desired.

3   Chill 1 hour. Use protein buns for sandwiches. Makes 8 servings.

NUTRITIONAL COMPARISON (PER SERVING)

TRADITIONAL SANDWICH = 445 CALORIES, 23G FAT, 27G PROTEIN, 30G CARBS, 2.4G CARBS

"HEALTHIFIED" SANDWICH = 325 CALORIES, 22G FAT, 29G PROTEIN, 4G CARBS, 1.5G FIBER (61% FAT, 35% PROTEIN, 5% CARBS)

"HEALTHIFIED" BURRITO

"TORTILLA"

Some coconut oil/butter/peanut oil for frying

3 eggs, separated

¼ cup Jay Robb's unflavored egg white or whey protein

2 oz cream cheese, softened (or egg yolks, if sensitive to dairy)

FILLING

2 cups organic lettuce

1 pound organic chicken/beef/pork loin

1 jar marinated peppers (or sautéed fresh peppers)

1 cup salsa

1 avocado

DIRECTIONS:

1   To make the "tortilla": Separate the eggs (save the yolks for a different recipe), and whip the whites in a clean, dry, cool bowl for a few minutes until very stiff. Blend in the whey protein. Slowly stir in the cream cheese (without breaking down the whites).

2   Heat the oil in a fry pan on medium-high heat until you can put a drop of water in and it will sizzle. Once it is hot, place a circle of dough (the "tortilla" mixture) on the pan. Fry until golden brown on both sides.

3   Remove from heat and place on a plate. Fill with your desired burrito filling and enjoy! Makes 4 servings.

NUTRITIONAL COMPARISON (PER SERVING)

CHIPOTLE TORTILLA = 290 CALORIES, 9G FAT, 7G PROTEIN, 44G CARBS, 2G FIBER

"HEALTHIFIED" TORTILLA = 126 CALORIES, 10G FAT, 10G PROTEIN, 1G CARB, TRACE FIBER

(68% FAT, 28% PROTEIN, 4% CARBS)

DORO WATT

INGREDIENTS:

2 large onions, finely chopped

1 clove garlic, minced

½ cup butter (or coconut oil/duck fat/leaf lard/beef tallow/bacon fat, if dairy sensitive)

4 tbsp organic Ethiopian Berbere

2 tsp Celtic sea salt

1 whole chicken, separated into legs, breasts, and thighs

8 organic hard boiled eggs

DIRECTIONS:

1   Chop the onions and place into a slow-cooker with the garlic and butter/oil, Berbere, and salt. Turn on low and let sit over night or until the onions caramelize.

2   In the morning (or after 8 hours), place the chicken into the slow-cooker and let it cook for another 8 hours or until the chicken is done and very tender.

3   Meanwhile, cook the hard boiled eggs. Place the chicken and onion mixture onto a beautiful dish and mix in the hard boiled eggs. *So* good and easy! Makes 8 servings.

NUTRITIONAL INFO (PER SERVING)

"HEALTHIFIED" DORO WATT = 315 CALORIES, 25G FAT, 19G PROTEIN, 4 CARBS, 0.8G FIBER (71% FAT, 24% PROTEIN, 5% CARBS)

DESSERTS

ANGEL FOOD CAKE WITH CUSTARD OR LEMON CURD

INGREDIENTS:

12 egg whites

2 tsp cream of tartar

1 pinch of salt

1 cup Jay Robb's strawberry protein powder (or egg white powder, if dairy sensitive)

1 cup Swerve Sweetener (Confectioners Style) or erythritol and 1 tsp stevia glycerite

1 tsp strawberry extract (or other extract)

LEMON CURD

1 cup Swerve Sweetener (Confectioners Style)

½ cup lemon juice

4 large eggs

1 tbsp finely grated lemon peel

8 tbsp coconut oil (or butter, if not dairy sensitive)

OPTIONAL CUSTARD

12 large egg yolks

1 cup unsweetened almond milk

½ cup Swerve Sweetener (Confectioners Style)

½ cup coconut oil (or butter), melted

DIRECTIONS:

1   Preheat oven to 350 degrees F. Sift whey protein and sweetener together and set aside. In a large clean bowl, whip egg whites with a pinch of salt until foamy (save the yolks for "healthified" crème brûlée, "healthified" coconut custard, or "healthified" ice cream). Add cream of tartar and continue to beat until very stiff (you will be able to put the bowl upside down and the whites won't fall out). Add your favorite extract flavor.

Quickly fold in whey mixture. Pour into a greased 10-inch tube pan. Bake at 350 degrees F for 45 minutes. Makes 14 servings. It also makes great French toast.

1   LEMON CURD: Combine natural sweetener, lemon juice, 4 eggs, and lemon peel in heavy, medium-sized saucepan and whisk to blend. Add butter. Whisk constantly over medium heat until mixture thickens and coats back of spoon thickly (do not boil) (about 12 minutes). Pour mixture through strainer into medium-sized bowl. Place bowl in larger bowl filled with ice water and whisk occasionally until lemon curd is cooled completely (about 15 minutes). Can be made 1 day ahead. Makes 12 servings.

1   CUSTARD (If you don't like lemon): Whisk egg yolks, almond milk, and sweetener in medium-sized metal bowl to blend. Slowly mix in the melted oil/butter so the eggs don't cook unevenly. Set bowl over saucepan of simmering water. Whisk mixture constantly and vigorously until thickened and the instant-read thermometer inserted into mixture registers 140 degrees F. Do this for about 3 to 5 minutes total (or until the mixture coats the back of a spoon). Remove the bowl the mixture is in from over the cold water. Serve warm or chilled. (If serving chilled, it can be prepared 1 to 3 days ahead and refrigerated. Re-whisk before serving.)

NUTRITIONAL INFO (PER SERVING)

TRADITIONAL ANGEL FOOD = 159 CALORIES, 0.7G FAT, 5.5G FIBER, 35G CARBS, 0.2G FIBER

"HEALTHIFIED" ANGEL FOOD = 54 CALORIES, 1G FAT, 11.1G PROTEIN, 0.9G CARBS, 0G FIBER
    (11% FAT, 82% PROTEIN, 7% CARBS)

"HEALTHIFIED" ANGEL FOOD WITH LEMON CURD =
    146 CALORIES, 10G FAT, 13G PROTEIN, 1G CARBS, TRACE FIBER
    (61% FAT, 36% PROTEIN, 3% CARBS)

KETO FUDGE

INGREDIENTS:

1 cup coconut oil, soft yet still solid

¼ cup full-fat coconut milk

¼ cup organic cocoa powder

¼ cup Swerve Sweetener (Confectioners Style)

1 tsp vanilla oil or extract

½ tsp almond oil extract

½ tsp Celtic sea salt

DIRECTIONS:

1   Place the coconut oil and coconut milk in a medium-sized bowl and mix with a hand mixer on high for 6 minutes or until well combined and glossy. TIP: I used my stand mixer.

2   Place the remaining ingredients in the bowl and stir on low speed until the cocoa is combined (so it doesn't poof all over your kitchen). Increase speed, and mix until everything is well combined. Taste the fudge and adjust to desired sweetness.

3   Place a sheet of parchment or wax paper along the inside of a loaf pan.

4   Pour fudge into loaf pan.

5   Place the loaf pan in the freezer for at least 15 minutes, until just set.

6   Use the edges of the parchment to pull the fudge out of the pan.

7   Place on a cutting board and remove the parchment paper.

8   Use a sharp knife to cut the fudge into squares.

9   Store in an airtight container in the freezer; it will liquefy if you leave it in a warm area. Makes 12 servings.

NUTRITIONAL INFO (PER SERVING)

TRADITIONAL FUDGE = 205 CALORIES, 19.6G FAT, 1G PROTEIN, 17G CARBS, 1G FIBER

"HEALTHIFIED" FUDGE = 172 CALORIES, 20G FAT, 1G PROTEIN, 1G CARBS, 0.6G FIBER (97% FAT, 0.9% PROTEIN, 2.1% CARBS)

FLOUR-LESS CHOCOLATE TORTE

INGREDIENTS:

7 oz unsweetened baking chocolate

14 tbsp (1 ¾ sticks) organic butter or coconut oil

1 ¼ cup Swerve Sweetener (Confectioners Style)

1 tbsp stevia glycerite (adjust to desired sweetness)

5 large eggs

1 tbsp coconut flour

DIRECTIONS:

1   Preheat oven to 375 degrees F. Grease an 8-inch pan and line with
    parchment paper (or use mini muffin tins). Grease parchment paper.
    Brown the butter (if desired … it tastes way better!) in a saucepan.
    Once the butter is brown (not black!), slowly add the chocolate (don't
    burn the chocolate). Add the sweetener. Mix well and let cool (in fridge
    to speed up the process). Once cool, add one egg at a time, mixing until
    well combined. Bake for 25 minutes. Serve with cream cheese frosting.
    Makes 10 servings.

NUTRITIONAL INFO (PER SERVING)   .

TRADITIONAL TORTE = 521 CALORIES, 27.4G FAT, 4.8G PROTEIN, 57G CARBS, 2.1G FIBER

"HEALTHIFIED" TORTE = 303 CALORIES, 31G FAT, 5G PROTEIN, 5G CARBS, 3G FIBER
(92% FAT, 5% PROTEIN, 5% CARBS)

MOLTEN CHOCOLATE CAKE

INGREDIENTS:

4 oz unsweetened baking chocolate

½ cup coconut oil

3 egg yolks

¼ to ½ cup Swerve Sweetener (Confectioners Style)

3 egg whites

DIRECTIONS:

1 Lightly grease 3 ramekins with butter. Melt the chocolate into the butter in a double boiler and let cool a bit.

2 Beat the egg yolks and natural sweetener and mix into the chocolate. Beat the egg whites in a bowl until they form soft peaks.

3 Fold the chocolate into the egg whites. Pour the batter into the ramekins, no more than ⅔ full.

4 Bake in a preheated 400 degrees F oven for 7 to 10 minutes. The outside will be set and will possibly crack, but the inside will still be liquid.

5 Let cool for a few minutes and then run a knife around the edges and tip onto a plate. (Optional: Feel free to eat it right out of the ramekin with a spoon.) Makes 3 servings.

NUTRITIONAL COMPARISON (PER SERVING)

TRADITIONAL CAKE = 488 CALORIES, 27G FAT, 7G PROTEIN, 55G CARBS, 3G FIBER

"HEALTHIFIED" CAKE = 577 CALORIES, 60G FAT, 11G PROTEIN, 11G CARBS, 5G FIBER (91% FAT, 7% PROTEIN, 3% CARBS)

MORE HIGH FAT AND MODERATE PROTEIN IDEAS

FRIED CHICHARRONES WITH GUACAMOLE

BRAUNSCHWEIGER (LIVERWURST)

CRACKLINGS

SAUSAGES (PORK AND LIVER)

LIVER AND ONIONS (RICH IN SULFUR)

•

30 DAY MEAL PLANS

In an ideal day, you would include intermittent fasting and exercise. I have designed an in depth 30 day meal plans that are keto-adapted and dairy free to get you healing quickly and losing weight fast. They include 30 detailed daily meal plans, weekly summaries with full grocery lists, over a dozen instructional videos and much more. To get started, just go here:

mariamindbodyhealth.com/my-services

I found Maria in April of 2012, in my 2nd semester of graduate school (which was when the photo of my "before" picture was taken). My mom had sent me a link to her blog, and I immediately started trying her recipes. Shortly after, I decided to take her health assessment and started a diet plan and taking the supplements she had suggested. Before the "Maria Way" I was eating over 100 grams of carbohydrates a day and who knows how much sugar. I experienced intense hunger and mood swings when my blood sugar would drop between meals. In less than a week of eating the Maria Way, I longer had fluctuations in my blood sugar, and as

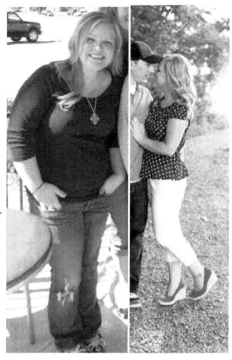

a result, I could think clearer! But then the stress of graduate school kicked in, and I began returning to my old eating habits. In January of 2013, I attempted to start eating the Maria Way again and even joined a gym. I've lost 25 pounds since January, and with my upcoming wedding I am working hard to meet my weight loss goals. I still struggle sticking to the diet on the weekends, but I hope to update Maria with my "after" photo this spring!

—Emily

Chapter 11

Summary

Maria, I have struggled with weight loss my entire life since I was six years old and my doctor put me on my first low-fat and low-calorie diet. I would lose 5 pounds here and there but remained heavy. As a kid, it is hard to stay on a restrictive diet because the first time you are allowed anything sweet you eat all that you can because you have been deprived of it for so long. Time passed, and when I was in 7th grade, my mom decided to try out the Atkins diet that helped me succeed in my weight loss, taking off 60 pounds in about 15 months. I had never felt better and really kept it off until I got my first job at a fast food restaurant when I was seventeen. The weight started coming back after a few too many fries, and then I was eating fast food nearly everyday at work and gaining despite living an active lifestyle.

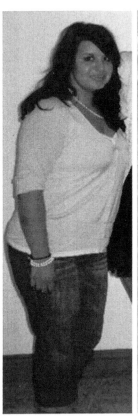
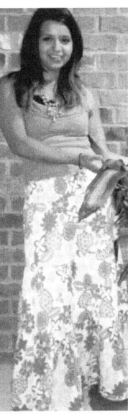

The years passed and I steadily gained at 145 pounds (at 5'2). My doctor had suggested I start trying to lose weight, as my blood sugar was very unbalanced and my blood pressure was abnormally high for a 20-year-old. I was starting to have the problems of a 50-year-old at the age of 20.

When I was 23, I found out my husband and I were pregnant and I stopped all dieting and ate whatever, whenever, and a lot of it. I had a nightmare of a pregnancy, being put on bed rest for high blood pressure at 4 months along. At the time of delivery, I was 207 pounds. I was so unhealthy and completely miserable; fighting off cravings was nearly impossible and my weight had gotten out of control. After the baby and things started to settle, I once again reached towards a low-carb lifestyle. It was harder this time after consuming so much junk food for years to go back to low-carb eating. At that time I didn't realize there were low-carb desserts and had never heard of my beloved almond flour. Even though I was low-carbing during the week, I would allow myself junk food on the weekend. Needless to say, my progress was very slow and disappointing and I fell off the low-carb wagon.

In November 2011, after bad blood work revealing I was prediabetic and my blood pressure was once again going up, I decided I really had to make a change in my life. I decided that this time I was going to take a different approach to low carb and really seek out recipes so that I wouldn't feel deprived. Pinterest had just started up at the time, so I pinned low-carb desserts by a blogger named Maria Emmerich, who single-handedly changed everything I ever thought about nutrition, dieting, and living a healthy lifestyle. I began buying the ingredients she suggested and making her recipes, which left me feeling amazing and satisfied. One month in and I was down 15 pounds! I couldn't believe it, I was eating all these great foods and losing, I never hit a plateau, and even started incorporating exercise into my life. When I first started living the "Maria Way," I was 170 pounds; one year later I was 115 pounds. I couldn't believe I had lost 55 pounds in one year! The best part was when I went to the doctor and they didn't even recognize me. It was the best feeling ever. My doctor was surprised at my appearance, but did warn that my blood work may not be any different because the low-carb lifestyle promotes high fat (blah, blah, yawn). Well, did I prove him wrong: my blood pressure was perfect and my prediabetes was gone. The doctor left saying, "Well, you have cured yourself. You are in perfect health."

I have been living the "Maria Way" for nearly two years now and I have never been happier! You have changed my life, the way I look at food, and have inspired me more than you could ever know. Everyday I am thankful for you in my life because without you, this would not have been possible.

—Amanda

So with all of the information I have provided you in this book, I wish you luck in your journey to a healthy weight and to a body that is healed from whatever ails you. I know this may all seem overwhelming and new, but rip off that Band-Aid. No more deprivation diets of fat-free, man-made foods … You need real food, real satisfaction, and a healthy mind and body.

Steps to Remember:

1. Add more medium-chain fats, like coconut oil, macadamia nut oil, and organic butter (if not dairy sensitive).

2. Add in a teaspoon of cinnamon at each meal to lower insulin response.

3. Add quality salt to your diet.

4. Drink homemade bone broth to eliminate dehydration, headaches, and muscle cramps.

5. Potassium

6. Magnesium

7. Calcium

8. Exercise in a fasted state.

And, just because I love them so much, here is my happy, healthy keto family.

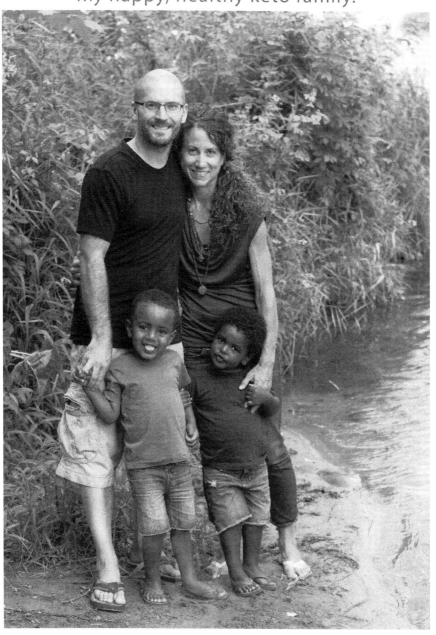

Notes

[1] "Our brains, for instance, are 70 percent fat, mostly in the form of a substance known as myelin that insulates nerve cells and, for that matter, all nerve endings in the body. Fat is the primary component of all cell membranes. Changing the proportion of saturated to unsaturated fats in the diet, as proponents of Keys's hypothesis recommended, might well change the composition of the fats in the cell membranes. This could alter the permeability of cell membranes, which determines how easily they transport, among other things, blood sugar, proteins, hormones, bacteria, viruses, and tumor-causing agents into and out of the cell." Gary Taubes, *Good Calories, Bad Calories* (New York: Anchor, 2008), p. 30–31.

[2] "Fat is also preferred by our nervous systems. Without fat, our neurotransmitters literally can't transmit. Twenty-five percent of the body's cholesterol is in the brain, the brain that is made up of over 60 percent saturated fat. The brain's glial cells play a primary role in cognitive function: they provide 'a substance that allows … synapses to form, and function. Without this substance your brain would be almost entirely useless.' The name of this wonder substance? Cholesterol." Lierre Keith, *The Vegetarian Myth*, p. 182.

[3] H. Takeuchi, S. Sekine, K. Kojima, and T. Aoyama, "The application of medium-chain fatty acids: edible oil with a suppressing effect on body fat accumulation," *Asia Pacific Journal of Clinical Nutrition* 17, no. 1 (2008): 320–3, http://www.ncbi.nlm.nih.gov/pubmed/18296368.

[4] M-P. St-Onge and P.J.H. Jones, "Greater rise in fat oxidation with medium-chain triglyceride consumption relative to long-chain triglyceride is associated with lower initial body weight and greater loss of subcutaneous adipose tissue," *International Journal of Obesity* 27, no. 12 (2003): 1565–1571, doi:10.1038/sj.ijo.0802467.

[5] Nutrition Review: Medium Chain Triglycerides (MCTs) "Nourishing Traditions"; Sally Fallon with Mary G. Enig, PhD; 2000

[6] "Plasma protein glycation in Alzheimer's disease," http://www.ncbi.nlm.nih.gov/pubmed/10211709.

[7] "Gluconeogenesis and energy expenditure after a high-protein, carbohydrate-free diet," http://ajcn.nutrition.org/content/90/3/519.full.pdf.

[8] Lierre Keith, *The Vegetarian Myth*, p.182.

[9] "Could Sulfur Deficiency be a Contributing Factor in Obesity, Heart Disease, Alzheimer's and Chronic Fatigue Syndrome?" http://people.csail.mit.edu/seneff/sulfur_obesity_alzheimers_muscle_wasting.html.

[10] Bonnie J. Brehm et al., "A Randomized Trial Comparing a Very Low Carbohydrate Diet and a Calorie-Restricted Low Fat Diet on Body Weight and Cardiovascular Risk Factors in Healthy Women," *Journal of Clinical Endocrinology & Metabolism* 88, no. 4 (2003): 1617,http://jcem.endojournals.org/content/88/4/1617.long.

[11] "A low-carbohydrate diet is more effective in reducing body weight than healthy eating in both diabetic and non-diabetic subjects," http://onlinelibrary.wiley.com/doi/10.1111/j.1464-5491.2007.02290.x/abstract.

[12] "Beneficial effects of ketogenic diet in obese diabetic subjects," http://link.springer.com/article/10.1007%2Fs11010-007-9448-z.

[13] "Long-term effects of a very-low-carbohydrate weight loss diet compared with an isocaloric low-fat diet after 12 months," http://ajcn.nutrition.org/content/90/1/23.long.

[14] "Carbohydrate Restriction has a More Favorable Impact on the Metabolic Syndrome than a Low Fat Diet," http://link.springer.com/article/10.1007%2Fs11745-008-3274-2.

[15] "Separate effects of reduced carbohydrate intake and weight loss on atherogenic dyslipidemia," http://ajcn.nutrition.org/content/83/5/1025.long.

[16] "Comparison of the Atkins, Zone, Ornish, and LEARN Diets for Change in Weight and Related Risk Factors Among Overweight Premenopausal Women," http://jama.jamanetwork.com/article.aspx?articleid=205916.

[17] "Short-term effects of severe dietary carbohydrate-restriction advice in Type 2 diabetes," http://onlinelibrary.wiley.com/doi/10.1111/j.1464-5491.2005.01760.x/abstract.

[18] "Efficacy and Safety of a High Protein, Low Carbohydrate Diet for Weight Loss in Severely Obese Adolescents," http://www.ncbi.nlm.nih.gov/pmc/articles/PMC2892194/.

[19] "Eating More Meals Does NOT Speed Up Your Metabolism," http://www.theiflife.com/eating-more-meals-does-not-speed-up-your-metabolism/.

[20] "Aging and Metabolism," http://www.innovitaresearch.org/news/06101801.html.

[21] "Minerals and phytic acid interactions: Is it a real problem for human nutrition?" http://onlinelibrary.wiley.com/doi/10.1046/j.1365-2621.2002.00618.x/full.

[22] "Reduced plasma half-life of radio-labelled 25-hydroxyvitamin D3 in subjects receiving a high-fibre diet," http://www.ncbi.nlm.nih.gov/pubmed/6299329.

[23] "The Ketogenic Diet as a Treatment Paradigm for Diverse Neurological Disorders," http://www.ncbi.nlm.nih.gov/pmc/articles/PMC3321471/.

[24] "Debunking Constipation Myths: The Truth About High Fiber Diets And Laxatives," http://www.sciencedaily.com/releases/2005/01/050111122655.htm.

[25] "First Genetic Link to Common Migraine Exposed," *Physorg.com*, Aug. 29, 2010, http://www.physorg.com/news202139760.html.

[26] David N. Ruskin and Susan A. Masino, "The Nervous System and Metabolic Dysregulation: Emerging Evidence Converges on Ketogenic Diet Therapy," Front Neurosci 6 (2012): 33, doi:10.3389/fnins.2012.00033.

[27] Dr. Richard Johnson, *The Fat Switch*

[28] Jo Robinson, *Eating on the Wild Side*

[29] Robert Lustig, *Fat Chance: Beating the Odds Against Sugar, Processed Food, Obesity, and Disease*

[30] Bruce Fife, *Stop Alzheimer's Now*

[31] Elaine Schmidt, "This is your brain on sugar: UCLA study shows high-fructose diet sabotages learning, memory; Eating more omega-3 fatty acids can offset damage, researchers say," *UCLA Newsroom*, 12 May 2012, http://newsroom.ucla.edu/portal/ucla/this-is-your-brain-on-sugar-ucla-233992.aspx.

[32] Hilary Parker, "A sweet problem: Princeton researchers find that high-fructose corn syrup prompts considerably more weight gain," *News at Princeton*, 22 March 2010, http://www.princeton.edu/main/news/archive/S26/91/22K07/.

[33] Duke Medicine News and Communications, "Increased Fructose Consumption May Deplete Cellular Energy in Patients with Obesity and Diabetes," 2 May 2012, http://www.dukehealth.org/health_library/news/increased-fructose-consumption-may-deplete-cellular-energy-in-patients-with-obesity-and-diabetes.

[34] Laura Gabriela Sánchez-Lozada, MyPhuong Le, Mark Segal and Richard J Johnson, "How safe is fructose for persons with or without diabetes?" *American Journal of Clinical Nutrition* 88, no. 5 (2008): 1189-1190, http://ajcn.nutrition.org/content/88/5/1189.full.

[35] A. Gul, M.A. Rahman, S.N. Hasnain, "Role of fructose concentration on cataractogenesis in senile diabetic and non-diabetic patients," *Graefe's Archive for Clinical and Experimental Ophthalmology* 247, no. 6 (2009): 809-14, doi:10.1007/s00417-008-1027-9.

[36] Andrew Schneider, "Tests Show Most Store Honey Isn't Honey: Ultra-filtering Removes Pollen, Hides Honey Origins," *Food Safety News*, 7 November 2011, http://www.foodsafetynews.com/2011/11/tests-show-most-store-honey-isnt-honey/#.UiCEVz94yGd.

[37] Lance Devon, "Seventy-five percent of honey bought at the supermarket isn't real honey," *Natural News.com*, 28 May 2013, http://www.naturalnews.com/040520_honey_supermarkets_counterfeit_food.html#ixzz2dS51AidW.

[38] http://nutritiondata.self.com/facts/sweets/5568/2

[39] "Nutritional and Health Benefits of Coconut Sap Sugar/Syrup,"

http://www.pca.da.gov.ph/coconutrde/images/sugarpdfs/TPTrinidad_FNRI.pdf

[40] M. Kim, H.K. Shin, "The water-soluble extract of chicory reduces glucose uptake from the perfused jejunum in rats," *Journal of Nutrition* 126, no. 9 (1996): 2236-42, http://www.ncbi.nlm.nih.gov/pubmed/8814212.

[41] "Sugar components of coconut sugar in Indonesia," http://www.cabdirect.org/abstracts/19930319960.html;jsessionid=275098A04771FE19A14BD4EAB1A-FA261.

[42] http://articles.mercola.com/sites/articles/archive/2010/03/30/beware-of-the-agave-nectar-health-food.aspx#_edn1.

[43] "Cotton Candy Grapes Are Seriously Sweet," http://m.neatorama.com/2013/08/08/Cotton-Candy-Grapes-Are-Seriously-Sweet/#!h3ezN

[44] "Breeding the Nutrition Out of Our Food," http://www.nytimes.com/2013/05/26/opinion/sunday/breeding-the-nutrition-out-of-our-food.html?pagewanted=all&_r=0.

[45] "Dietary fructose reduces circulating insulin and leptin, attenuates postprandial suppression of ghrelin, and increases triglycerides in women," http://www.ncbi.nlm.nih.gov/pubmed/15181085.

[46] http://umm.edu/health/medical/altmed/supplement/lysine

[47] Jeff S. Volek, PhD, RD and Stephen D. Phinney, MD, PhD, *The Art and Science of Low Carbohydrate Performance* (Beyond Obesity LLC, 2012).

[48] Natan Gadoth and Hans Hilmar Göbel, eds. *Oxidative Stress and Free Radical Damage in Neurology*, (Mainz: Humana Press, 2011),p. 37–39.

[49] "Start running and watch your brain grow, say scientists," http://www.theguardian.com/science/2010/jan/18/running-brain-memory-cell-growth.

[50] "The Ketogenic Diet," http://www.health-matrix.net/2013/08/09/the-ketogenic-diet-an-overview/.

[51] "Celiac Disease-Associated Autoimmune Endocrinopathies," http://cvi.asm.org/content/8/4/678.full.

[52] "Is celiac disease a wheat allergy?" http://celiacdisease.about.com/od/whatisceliacdisease/f/AllergyVsAutoim.htm.

[53] "Strict adherence for life is essential," http://www.cureceliacdisease.org/medical-professionals/guide/treatment.

[54] "Is fibromyalgia an autoimmune disorder of endogenous vasoactive neuropeptides?" http://www.ncbi.nlm.nih.gov/pubmed/15082086.

[55] David N. Ruskin and Susan A. Masino, "The Nervous System and Metabolic Dysregulation: Emerging Evidence Converges on Ketogenic Diet Therapy," *Frontiers in Neuroscience*, 6 (2012): 33, doi: 0.3389/fnins.2012.00033.

[56] http://articles.mercola.com/sites/articles/archive/2011/06/19/innovative-revolutionary-program-to-keep-your-body-biologically-young.aspx.

[57] Jeff S. Volek, PhD, RD and Stephen D. Phinney, MD, PhD, *The Art and Science of Low Carb Living* (Beyond Obesity LLC, 2011), p. 35.

[58] "Alcohol concentration and carbonation of drinks: the effect on blood alcohol levels," http://www.ncbi.nlm.nih.gov/m/pubmed/17720590/.

[59] Jimmy Moore and Eric C. Westman, MD, *Cholesterol Clarity*, (Victory Belt Publishing, 2013).

38163139R00155

Printed in Great Britain
by Amazon